Community Health Nursing:
A CASE STUDY APPROACH

Community Health Nursing:

A CASE STUDY APPROACH

Tamara Hertenstein McKinnon, RN, MSN
Lecturer and Clinical Instructor
San Jose State University
San Jose, California

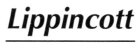

Lippincott

Philadelphia • New York

Acquisitions Editor: Susan M. Glover, RN, MSN
Project Editor: Gretchen Metzger
Production Manager: Helen Ewan
Production Coordinator: Patricia McCloskey
Design Coordinator: Melissa Olson
Indexer: Alexandra Nickerson

9   8   7   6   5   4   3   2   1

Library of Congress Cataloging in Publications Data
Hertenstein-McKinnon, Tamara.
   Community health nursing: a case study approach/Tamara
   Hertenstein McKinnon.
      p.   cm.
   Includes bibliographical references and index.
   ISBN 0–397–55460–5 (alk. paper)
   1. Community health nursing.   I. Title
   DNLM: 1. Community Health Nursing. WY 106 H573c 1997
RT98.H47   1997
610.73'43—DC20   96–41028
DNLM/DLC
for Library of Congress   CIP

Care has been taken to confirm the accuracy of the information presented and to describe generally accepted practices. However, the authors, editors, and publisher are not responsible for errors or omissions or for any consequences from application of the information in this book and make no warranty, express or implied, with respect to the contents of the publication.

The authors, editors, and publisher have exerted every effort to ensure that drug selection and dosage set forth in this text are in accordance with current recommendations and practice at the time of publication. However, in view of ongoing research, changes in government regulations, and the constant flow of information relating to drug therapy and drug reactions, the reader is urged to check the package insert for each drug for any change in indications and dosage and for added warnings and precautions. This is particularly important when the recommended agent is a new or infrequently employed drug.

Some drugs and medical devices presented in this publication have Food and Drug Administration (FDA) clearance for limited use in restricted research settings. It is the responsibility of the health care provider to ascertain the FDA status of each drug or device planned for use in their clinical practice.

This book is dedicated
with love and appreciation
to my wonderful husband David
and to our sons Aaron and Lucas.

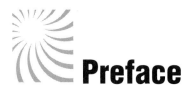 **Preface**

The goal of this text is to afford learners, both nursing students and practicing nurses, an opportunity to develop critical thinking skills in the area of community health nursing. The cases presented in this text are intended to provoke the learner—to stimulate thoughtful discussion and introspection. There is no single correct response to exercises or case studies. With feedback from instructors and peers, learners will add to their repertoire while identifying areas warranting further study.

The text provides an historical overview of community health nursing and analyzes trends in health care that have influenced and will continue to influence nursing practice. The emphasis of this text is on analysis of key concepts of community health nursing: the skills and theoretical knowledge base needed for professional practice in the community setting. Theoretical concepts are presented along with a corresponding discussion of their functional applications. Case studies and exercises allow learners to apply community health nursing principles to situations with varying degrees of complexity. The topics covered will command learners' attention because they are relevant, timely, and realistic.

Learners, working in pairs or groups, will learn from one another about relevant community health issues. They will prepare for intervention in the community by researching data related to diagnosis, practice setting, and psychosocial conditions. This text may be used alone or in conjunction with any current community health nursing textbook. Other resources that will assist learners in working through case studies and exercises include community resource directories and textbooks from other areas of nursing practice, ie, obstetrics, medical-surgical, and psychiatric.

Until recently, students in community health nursing practicums as well as new community health nurses have been trained by nurses working in a specific area of practice. Although this type of mentorship remains invaluable, the addition of thousands of new nursing positions in diverse community health settings limits its application. There is a real need for nurses and nursing students to be introduced to relevant and timely scenarios dealing with current health care issues in diverse community health nursing settings, with clients whose psychosocial issues are representative of those facing today's population. This text is designed to fill those educational and training needs.

The unique feature of this book is its presentation of cases that deal with current issues affecting clients in their environment of care. This approach will challenge learners to problem solve cases using knowledge gained from community health nursing theories and drawing upon general nursing knowledge.

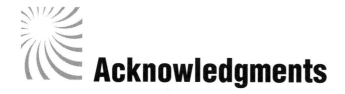

Acknowledgments

I would like to thank Carol Huston who has given unselfishly of her valuable time and expertise. I am honored to have a mentor who personifies professionalism in nursing.

Dr. Jean Sullivan, Barbara Moberly, Suzanne Grant, and Tracy Baucom are community health nurses whose input was invaluable in the preparation of the text.

This book would not have been possible without the support and encouragement that I received from individuals at the following agencies: Santa Cruz County Health Services Agency, in particular the staff of California Childrens' Services; Prime Health at Home; and San Jose State and Sacramento State Universities' School of Nursing.

The editorial staff at Lippincott-Raven Publishers, most notably Susan Glover, demonstrated remarkable flexibility in the development of this text.

I would like to express my appreciation to the families who open their homes and their hearts to nurses working in the community. Their willingness to share information about their lives is a constant source of inspiration.

Special thanks to my family and friends, especially Kathy and Jon Powell, Trish Harris, Mike Hertenstein, Ed and Edith Hertenstein, Kerry Carpenter, the Lupfers, Ann Farrier, and Martina Nicholson. And to Lou, who encouraged me to dare to dream.

Photo credits

David McKinnon and Kathy Powell

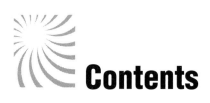 **Contents**

Community Health Nursing:

A CASE STUDY APPROACH

Introduction

CHAPTER FORMAT

The text contains 12 chapters, each focusing on a critical aspect of community health nursing practice. Each chapter is divided into three sections: review, discussion, and case studies and exercises. Chapters 1 through 3 provide an overview of current information related to the role of the community health nurse. Chapters 4 through 12 are organized by key concepts. These theories and principles are at the core of effective community nursing practice. Learners will use presented theories and principles as they respond to the cases and exercises.

Review

This section presents a synopsis, in outline form, of key concepts related to the chapter's topic. This overview provides the learner an opportunity to ensure a knowledge base sufficient for working through the exercises and case studies. Detailed information related to the outlined material may be obtained by reviewing supporting texts such as community health theory textbooks.

Discussion

This section presents a narrative overview of selected aspects of the chapter's topic.

Case Studies and Exercises

The intent of the case studies and exercises is to develop critical thinking skills specific to the practice of community health nursing. Cases are written in first person format and are representative of the multiple, complex issues facing today's community health nurses. Exercises and case studies are meant to provide the learner with ideas for addressing various issues.

Preparing responses for cases will simulate learners' preparation for actual community health visits. Personal reflection about responses to exercises and cases, along with feedback from peers and instructors, will guide the learner in the development of skills and knowledge related to professional community health nursing practice.

Regarding institutions for which terminology may vary by region, for example, Medicaid, Children's Protective Services, and Public Health Department, an effort has been made to use generic terms.

APPLICATION

Teaching and Learning Strategies. Both case studies and exercises may be worked through in any of the following ways. Case studies are flexible and may be addressed by individuals, pairs, and small or large groups. Individuals and groups may use supporting texts when working through case studies and exercises.

Individual
1. Responses are reviewed by instructor, and feedback provided to learner.
2. Learner uses self reflection as a means of personal feedback.

Pair
1. "Ice breaker"
2. Sharing of personal or intimate responses
3. Sharing information between learners with varied areas of expertise
4. Working together, using each participant's area of expertise to address a problem or issue

Small group (2–4 people) or large group (5–8 people)
1. Team approach to problem resolution
2. Learners write responses (anonymously) and place in central location; instructor or selected class member reads responses aloud.
3. Information and personal responses shared within group
    If each group works through the same exercise or case:
    - Sharing information with other groups
    - Learning from other groups' responses to the cases and exercises
    - Analyzing variations in groups' responses
    If each group works through a different exercise or case:
    - Sharing information, including rationale for responses, with other groups
    - Obtaining feedback from other groups

Role Play
1. Learners assume roles and improvise based on information provided or personal interpretation of characters.
2. Scenario is acted out in front of class.

Debate
1. Groups are assigned opinions that they work together to defend.

Visualization
1. Facilitator reads exercise to group, lights are dimmed, and learners sit quietly with eyes closed and reflect on personal responses to exercise.

REFERENCE MAP INFORMATION

Cities on this factitious map will be referenced in exercises and case studies. Certain demographic information about the areas is presented below.

Smithville
Population: 4900
Employment: Agriculture (corn and wheat), seasonal variations
Schools: Two elementary, one combined junior high/high school
Services: Library, post office, public pool, three churches, Boys Club, no hospital

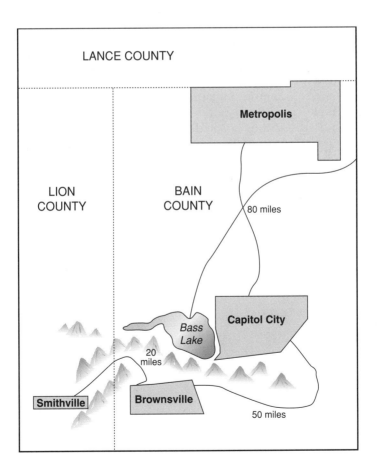

Brownsville

Population: 32,000

Employment: Manufacturing, agriculture-related businesses such as food processing, small Army base

Schools: Six elementary schools, three junior high schools, two high schools, and one junior college

Services: One small community hospital, community center with recreation programs, two public pools, three post offices, two libraries, YMCA/YWCA

Capitol City

Population: 98,000

Employment: Industry, manufacturing, education, and government

Schools: Sixteen elementary schools, one elementary/junior high school combined (private), six junior highs, four public and one private high school, one junior college and one state college

Services: Many governmental agencies, two large hospitals, extensive Parks and Recreation programs, four libraries, numerous churches and synagogues

Metropolis

Population: 262,000

Employment: Technology, manufacturing, government, education, and tourism

Schools: Numerous public and private elementary, junior high, and high schools; one junior college; and one university

Services: Teaching hospital affiliated with the university; numerous diverse places of worship; Parks and Recreation programs including elder day care; numerous libraries, community centers, and public pools

PART

I

OVERVIEW

CHAPTER 1

Evolving and Emerging Roles in Community-Based Nursing Practice

Whene'er a noble deed is wrought
Whene'er is spoke a noble thought
Our hearts, in glad surprise,
To higher levels rise.

The tidal wave of deeper souls
Into our inmost being rolls
And lifts us unawares
Out of all meaner cares.

Honor to those whose words or deeds
Thus help us in our daily needs.
And by their overflow
Raise us from what is low!

From: 'Santa Filomena' (Saint Florence)
by Henry Wadsworth Longfellow

To appreciate the direction that the field of community health nursing is taking, it is important to recognize its past. This chapter provides a review of the roots of community health nursing and addresses both 'traditional' (evolving) roles as well as emerging roles in community health. Specific functions and responsibilities of various specialty areas are highlighted in the Discussion.

REVIEW

I. Historical perspective
   A. Then: provision of district nursing care to the impoverished and infirmed
   B. Now: primary, secondary, and tertiary prevention to individuals, aggregates, and communities
II. Conceptual frameworks
   A. Theories
   B. Theorists
III. Research
   A. Historical
   B. Current
   C. Future
IV. Education
   A. Preparation for community health nursing practice
   B. Levels of practice
   C. Entry to practice
   D. Specialty areas
V. Traditional community health nursing roles
   A. Public health nurse
   B. Home health nurse
   C. Occupational health nurse
   D. School nurse
   E. Detention nurse

DISCUSSION

Evolving Roles in Community-Based Nursing Practice

PUBLIC HEALTH NURSING

A century ago, Lillian Wald created the concept of public health nursing. She defined it as "the link between families' social, economic, and health needs and the services that they required to get or stay well" (Buhler-Wilkerson, 1994, p. 327). Although the scope of practice of the public health nurse has seen dramatic changes in recent years, the basic tenets of public health nursing remain unchanged.

Implementation of public health principles is changing hands with reform of the health care system. In 1993 the American Public Health Association proposed "to transfer most of the personal clinical services provided by local health departments to health plans, while strengthening the population-based services" (Zerwekh, 1993, p. 328). Examples of this approach include school- and community-based clinic services and county-operated managed care systems.

Historically, public health nursing has been synonymous with district nursing. District, or field nurses, were responsible for the health concerns of the population living within their geographic territory. Although this approach provided holistic services to clients, demonstrating its cost effectiveness proved difficult. Consequently, use of this model has diminished in favor of more cost- and funding-based approaches.

Currently, most public health nursing positions are paid for, at least partially, by specific programs. This is referred to as "categorical funding." As a result of categorical funding, nurses' activities are dictated by the goals of these programs. Programs are designed to meet the health needs of the community by addressing specific, well-documented, identified health concerns. Examples of such programs include immunizations, communicable diseases, acquired immunodeficiency syndrome (AIDS), sexually transmitted diseases (STDs), health education, maternal health, children's health, tuberculosis, senior health, handicapped children, dental health, high-risk infant follow-up, substance use, and family planning. Most health departments also offer low- or no-cost clinic services to the communities they serve. This may include general medical clinics as well as specialty clinics such as family planning, immunization, tuberculosis, and AIDS and STD clinics.

Many health departments have affiliations with other agencies such as hospitals, long-term care facilities, and home health agencies. These affiliations have diminished due to competition from insurance companies such as health maintenance organizations (HMOs) and managed care organizations.

As a result of funding changes, today's public health nurses focus on populations whose commonality is the fact that they meet the criteria of a program that is funded to serve a specific aggregate, such as substance-using pregnant women or clients exposed to communicable diseases, rather than a population living within a particular geographic area. It is the responsibility of all public health nurses, particularly leaders in public health such as program managers and nursing directors, to identify needs of the community as a whole and to solicit funding for programs that will respond to those needs.

HOME HEALTH NURSING

Home health nursing is making a comeback with the rising cost of hospitalization and the aging of the American populace. "The segment of population older than 65 years will see rapid growth as it increases from fewer than 12% of the total population today to 21% in the year 2030" (Dansky, 1995, p. 15). In addition to demographic factors, technologic advances are redefining the practice of home health. Portable technology has made the provision of care in the home less expensive and more convenient for clients. Additionally, anecdotal information suggests that clients generally feel more comfortable receiving care in the home environment and consequently may experience better outcomes. As a result of these factors, home health agencies are rapidly replacing hospitals as the predominant employer of professional nurses.

Examples of areas in which home health nursing is expanding include prenatal home monitoring, postpartum home visitation, infusion therapy, high-risk infant follow-up, psychiatric care, and care for the technology (ie, ventilator) dependent. Home health nursing service continues to demonstrate good outcomes and cost effectiveness. An example of such cost effectiveness is a study that examined low birth weight infants discharged early, with visits from expert nurse clinicians. The results of this investigation indicated an average cost saving of over $18,000 per early discharge (Bednash, 1994, p. 84).

SCHOOL NURSING

The practice area for school nurses spans from elementary school to the university setting. Many of those who grew up before the 1980s can remember "their" school nurse. The school nurse was present on campus when school was in session and could help students with anything from a case of the stomach flu or a sore throat to providing a note to be excused from gym class. The school nurse also used expert knowledge of communicable diseases to address issues such as tuberculosis and head lice.

As with other community nursing roles, the role of the school nurse has changed, in great part because of economic constraints and societal influence. Although the traditional school nurse served a valuable purpose and intervened to make positive changes in the lives of children and their families, the cost effectiveness of these services was difficult to prove. Societal issues have entered the schools and are becoming a primary focus for school nurses. Examples of issues faced by today's school nurses include drug use, violence, teen (and preteen) pregnancy, STDs, family planning, and abortion. Family issues such as abuse, poverty, and mental illness may significantly influence students' lives and consequently become issues for the school nurse to address.

At a time when societal and family issues are affecting children as never before, the availability of school nurses is diminishing because of fiscal constraints. Fortunately, nurses are taking political action to address these issues and have demonstrated their importance in terms of both outcomes for students and cost effectiveness for taxpayers. As a result, some areas are experiencing regrowth, albeit slow, in the area of school nursing.

OCCUPATIONAL HEALTH NURSING

Perhaps the area of community health nursing that has and will continue to experience the greatest change is that of occupational health. Although the field of occupational health nursing has always been influenced by the rise and fall of employment levels (Table 1-1), the current changes primarily result from health care reform combined with the technologic revolution in the workplace.

TABLE 1-1

Significant Historical Events for Occupational Health Nursing in the United States, 1911–1992

1911	Workers' compensation legislation enacted
1912	38 nurses employed by business firms
1913	Registry opened in Boston for nurses to work in factory emergency rooms
1914	World War I begins 60 firms offer industrial nursing services
1916	U.S. government encourages employee health in shipyards, factories, and mills by war material contracts
1918	1,213 nurses employed in 871 business firms
1929	Stock market crash, beginning of Depression
1930	3,189 nurses employed in industry and commerce
1941	Beginning of World War II 6,244 occupational health nurses estimated working
1942	American Association of Industrial Nurses (AAIN) founded
1943	12,838 industrial nurses registered, 11,220 nurses actively working in industrial jobs
1970	Occupational Safety and Health Act passed Dept. of Labor—enforces OSHA standards, conducts workplace inspections, maintains death and injury statistics NIOSH—develops education and research activities 20,000 nurses employed in occupational health settings
1974	American Board for Occupational Health Nurses gives first certification examination
1976	AAIN becomes American Association of Occupational Health Nurses
1984	DHHS survey estimates almost 23,000 occupational health nurses in U.S.
1992	AAOHN celebrates 50th anniversary with 12,500 members Estimated 23,000 practicing occupational health nurses in U.S.

From Wassell (1995), with permission.

Historically, occupational health nurses' responsibilities have included the administration of first aid, home visitation to workers and their families, health supervision, and health promotion. The role of the occupational health nurse is expanding to include review of workmen's compensation cases, workplace safety, first aid and cardiopulmonary resuscitation (CPR) education, injury and accident prevention (ie, ergonomics, stress reduction), and case management.

Case management is the primary method of health insurance cost containment for many companies. The definition and a discussion of various types of case management are discussed in Chapter 10. Occupational health nurses may provide direct service or case coordination for employees with workmen's compensation cases. Nurses work with individual employees to determine the course of action, given an injury or disability. Direct service to employee clients may involve retraining and alterations in the work environment. Service coordination allows the nurse to work with the employee and providers of care to identify goals and coordinate efforts toward achievement of identified goals. In addition to case coordination in workmen's compensation cases, occupational health nurses may work with the company's insurance provider in the coordination of medical care for employees.

DETENTION NURSING

Nurses have long been the providers of health care to incarcerated populations. With the rise in prison populations, the number of nurses employed in such facilities is rapidly increasing. Changes in the prison population have created new issues for nurses working with that aggregate. For example, inmates who previously would have been admitted to an acute care facility, such as those with active tuberculosis, are increasingly being cared for in detention settings. As with other community health nurses, these nurses assess the needs of their population and identify actual and potential problems. Detention nurses serve their population through group education, injury and disease prevention measures, and direct care.

Issues that significantly influence the provision of nursing care to the incarcerated include personal safety, violence, STDs, AIDS, substance abuse, overcrowding, and racial tensions. Detention nurses must evaluate their scope of responsibility in dealing with the complex issues facing incarcerated populations. Many legal and ethical issues arise for nurses working in this setting. Detention nurses must be adept at working under the constraints of multiple systems because clarification of issues involves both the health care system and the legal system.

FORENSIC NURSING

Forensic nursing is a rapidly growing field that involves such specialty areas as sexual assault nurse examiner, insurance investigator, and crime scene analyst. Nurses working in this field may be employed by hospitals, health departments, insurance companies, or law enforcement.

COMMUNITY AGENCIES

Nonprofit community agencies are branching out into the provision of health care to the populations they serve. An example of this phenomenon is Planned Parenthood clinics. Although these clinics have been exemplary in their provision of family planning and abortion services, they have been known for those services exclusively. Recently, Planned Parenthood clinics began providing prenatal and other health care services. This approach offers more holistic care for clients in an environment that many women feel is most responsive to their needs.

With the increase in provision of direct nursing care to clients, along with expansions of health programs, community agencies and clinics are in need of qualified community health nurses. Possession of skills such as cultural sensitivity, multilingual ability, program development, direct provision of services, coordination with payer sources, and program administration will assist nurses working in community agencies.

INSURANCE COMPANIES

Private insurance companies, including HMOs, are hiring community health nurses, such as nurse case managers, as they strive for increased quality and cost containment. Federal and local governments are likewise discovering the value of nursing in the management of clients' health care services. With a focus on the provision of quality health care in the most cost-efficient manner, the advent of managed care has created thousands of new community health nursing positions.

ADVANCED PRACTICE NURSES

The number of advanced practice nurses, including nurse practitioners, nurse midwives, and clinical nurse specialists, is on the rise. Currently, 19% of primary care practitioners in the United States are nurses (Aiken & Salmon, 1994, p. 325). Health maintenance organizations have used the services of advanced practice nurses for many years and their role is increasing with health care reform. Advanced practice nurses offer cost savings, quality care, and a high level of client satisfaction.

Concerns related to advanced practice nurses include regulation, licensing, and reimbursement. Theoretical basis for practice is another point of contention related to advanced practice nursing. Dr. Imogene King, nurse theorist, has stated "the nurse practitioner extended nursing into medicine and the clinical nurse specialist had an expanded nursing role" (Huch, 1995, p. 44). The expanded role of nurses in health care reform may assist the profession in coming to a consensus regarding issues of advanced practice.

HOSPICE

Hospice involves the work of an interdisciplinary team, which often includes family members, in the provision of palliative care, psychosocial support, and pain control for the terminally ill. Although the principles of hospice have existed for centuries, the current version of hospice was borne out of work by two physicians, Elizabeth Kübler-Ross and Dame Cicely Saunders (Gentile & Fello, 1990, p. 1). Hospice nurses provide care for the terminally ill (generally regarded as those having a life expectancy of 6 months or less). This care may be provided in the client's home, a group home, or an inpatient setting. Hospice nurses must have a high level of clinical competence and must posses excellent interpersonal communication skills.

Many insurance companies, including Medicaid and Medicare, appreciate the value of hospice programs and reimburse for their services. Similarly, managed care companies have identified hospice as an agency that can coordinate quality care in a cost-effective manner.

Examples of services provided in most hospice programs include:

Nursing care
Medical care
Medications
Therapy services (ie, physical, occupational, etc)
In-home supportive services
Respite care
Counseling services
    Grief counseling
    Postdeath counseling for families
Referrals
    Legal aid

PRIVATE PRACTICE (STRESS MANAGEMENT)

It was recently reported that about 60% of visits to primary physicians' offices are stress related (Benson, 1995). Examples of maladies that are linked to, and may be exacerbated by, stress include headaches, sleep disorders and disturbances, and pain (such as the pain associated with cancer and AIDS). Nurses practicing in the area of stress management are in a position to provide skilled care that may lead to:

- Improved outcomes by addressing the true etiology of these problems
- Lower costs by using the most cost-effective practitioner
- Avoidance of further stress-related health problems through the use of preventive measures such as wellness programs

Additional Emerging and Evolving Roles

Trends in society and health care have created, and will continue to create, new opportunities for nurses. Examples of such opportunities include:

Private clinics and outpatient centers
Rural health
Health planning
Research
Continuous quality improvement
Governmental programs
    Medicare and Medicaid
Politics
Continuing education
Case management
Program administration
Policy planning
Education
    Consumers
    Providers

Managed care entities
Nurses: technical skills
Facilitation for integration of public and private programs
Administration of managed care programs
Legislation for health care reform
Fiscal intermediaries
Legal experts
Funding analysis

Case Studies and Exercises

Responses to the following case studies and exercises reflect the ability to:

1. Identify personal and societal perceptions of nurses working in community settings.
2. Differentiate between responsibilities in various (acute and community) nursing roles.
3. Describe the role of the community health nurse.
4. Discuss appropriate community health nursing interventions given various scenarios.

1.1 EXERCISE

COMMUNITY HEALTH NURSE ROLES

Questions

1) Discuss your impressions of the following community health nurse roles before your nursing education:
   - School nurse

   - Home health nurse

   - Public health nurse

2) Discuss how your perception of the roles and responsibilities of these and other community health nurses has changed with your nursing education.

3) Why is it important that health care providers and the general public are aware of the various specialty areas in community health nursing?

4) Discuss ways to increase awareness and update the public's perception of the areas of practice and level of expertise of the community health nurse.

5) Speculate about potential opportunities for nurses working in the community given:
   - The aging of the American population

   - Increasing financial demands on health care resources

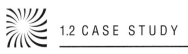 1.2 CASE STUDY

GERONTOLOGY

SCENARIO

Your client is Joseph, a 73-year-old man. Joseph experienced a myocardial infarction, along with a mild cerebrovascular accident (CVA), 10 days ago. He is being discharged from Capitol City Hospital to his home in

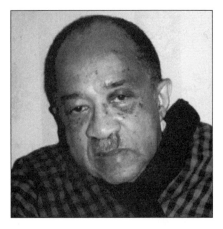

the suburbs of Capitol City. Joseph lives with his 66-year-old wife, Anna, who will be his primary caretaker. Anna enjoys good health and is "looking forward" to having her husband back home soon.

Questions

Discuss how your responsibilities in the care of Joseph may differ as you function in the nursing roles presented below.

1) RN in the medical-surgical unit of Capitol City Hospital

2) Discharge planner for Capitol City Hospital

3) PHN/Administrator of the Capitol City senior nutrition program

4) Home health nurse assigned Joseph's case

5) RN in Joseph's primary care physician's office

1.3 EXERCISE

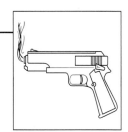

VIOLENCE

Questions

Violence is a major community health problem.

1) Discuss acts of violence affecting your community.

2) List five practice areas of community health nursing that might be involved in working to decrease violent activity in your community.

3) State ways in which these community health nurses are involved in attempts to reduce violence.

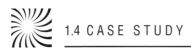 1.4 CASE STUDY

SEX EDUCATION

SCENARIO

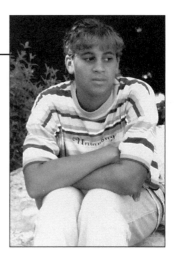

You are a school nurse working in a junior high school in Brownsville. A student, Andrea, approaches you one afternoon after school and asks if she can speak with you in private. Andrea tells you that her older sister recommended she speak with you about her concern. Andrea is 14 years old and has a steady boyfriend, Samuel. Samuel attends a local high school. Andrea and Samuel are sexually active. Andrea is concerned that she may become pregnant. "My friend told me that I couldn't get pregnant the first few times, Now that we've been 'doing it' for awhile I think maybe I could get pregnant, so my sister said to ask you for the pill or something."

The school board in Brownsville has a strict policy against the provision of birth control to minors. Your interpretation of this policy is that it is unacceptable to give birth control devices to students.

Questions

Consider your role as the school nurse. Discuss your approach to the following issues:

1) The possibility that Andrea may currently be pregnant.
   - How will you assess her pregnancy status?

- Where will you refer Andrea for follow-up (including birth control)?

2) Discuss means of education related to:
   - Birth control

   - STDs

3) Explore implications of dialogue, regarding sexual activity, with:
   - Andrea's boyfriend

   - Parents

4) How do these types of school nursing activities differ from those of the stereotypical school nurse?

1.5 EXERCISE

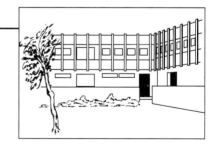

SEX EDUCATION SCHOOL POLICY

Note: Consider the scenario presented in Case Study 1.2.

Questions

1) If there is evidence that the school board's policy regarding education about contraception is having deleterious effects on the health of students, discuss ways that you, as the school nurse, will work to educate the school board, the general public, and school staff to effect necessary changes in the policy. Include a discussion of your personal

feelings and beliefs related to this issue and how they may influence your approach.

2) How involved should the school nurse be in this process? Explain your response.

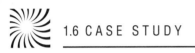

1.6 CASE STUDY

PEDIATRICS

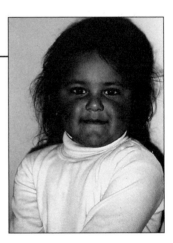

SCENARIO

You are a hospice nurse in Metropolis working with the family of a 6-year-old girl, Georgina, who has leukemia. Georgina was diagnosed as having acute lymphocytic leukemia (ALL) at age 3. No suitable bone marrow donor has been identified for her. Georgina was experiencing her second remission when she became ill 5 weeks ago. The pediatric oncologist advised the family that this relapse "does not look good," that Georgina's chances of long-term survival are quite low. She advised the family that Georgina's life expectancy is 4 to 6 months.

The physician encouraged the family to contact your hospice agency. You have the following information about the family:

The parents, Ron and Debbie, are divorced.

Ron lives in Capitol City where he works as a chef. He is remarried and has an 8-year-old stepson. Georgina stays with Ron every weekend and for extended periods during the summer.

Debbie works part-time, out of the home, as a seamstress. She has a large extended family in the area.

Georgina is an only child.

Question

1) Given the following actual or potential issues facing this family, discuss appropriate hospice nursing care services. In addition, identify possible

interdisciplinary resources that you, as the hospice nurse, will involve to ensure holistic care for this child and her family.

Issues (Actual and Potential)	Hospice Services	Ancillary Services (specify providers)
Psychological • Working through the stages of grief • Support groups • Stress reduction		
Social • Peer relationships		
Education • Health care • Disease process • Stages of death and dying		
Physiologic • Pain management • Fluid and nutritional needs • Risk of hemorrhage and infection		
Financial • Insurance • Family leave from employer • Funeral preparations		

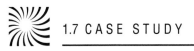 1.7 CASE STUDY

POLICIES AND STAFF EDUCATION

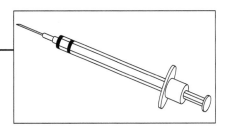

SCENARIO

As a nurse in the Capitol City jail, you provide direct care to inmates. One evening you observe a guard enter an inmate's cell and come out carrying an object. He heads to his supervisor's office and tosses the object in the trash can. Later, he tells you that what he found in the cell was intravenous (IV) drug "works," a syringe and needle. He says that he filed a report and that the occupants of the cell will be questioned about the paraphernalia.

Questions

1) What actual and potential problems can you identify from this scenario?

2) As a nurse in the jail, what are your responsibilities related to actual and potential problems?

1.8 EXERCISE

COMMUNITY HEALTH NURSE ROLES AND RESPONSIBILITIES

1) Discuss the roles and responsibilities that a community health nurse working in the following agencies might have:
   - Home health agency

   - Public health agency

   - School district

   - Migrant farm worker clinic

- Inner city volunteer center

- Large manufacturing firm

References

Aiken, L., & Salmon, M. (1994). Health care workforce priorities: What nursing should do now. *Inquiry, 31,* 318–329.

Bednash, G. (1994). The future of nursing and health care reform. Keynote speech 4/20/94. National Student Nurses Association. *NSNA/Imprint,* September/October, 83–85.

Benson, H. (1995, December 6). Harvard Medical School. *The Today Show.* New York: NBC.

Buhler-Wilkerson, K. (1994). Bringing care to the people: Lillian Wald's legacy to public health nursing. *American Journal of Public Health, 83,* 1778–1786.

Dansky, K. (1995). The impact of healthcare reform on rural home health agencies. *Journal of Nursing Administration, 25*(3), 27–33.

Gentile, M., & Fello, M. (1990). Hospice care for the 1990s: A concept coming of age. *Journal of Home Health Care Practice, 3*(1), 1–15.

Huch, M. (1995). Nursing and the next millennium. *Nursing Science Quarterly, 8*(1), 38–44.

Wassel, M. (1995). Occupational health nursing and the advent of managed care. *American Association of Occupational Health Nursing Journal, 43*(1), 23–28.

Zerwekh, J. V. (1993). Going to the people: Public health nursing today and tomorrow. *American Journal of Public Health, 83,* 1676–1678.

CHAPTER 2

Health Care Trends

"The farther backward you can look, the farther forward you are likely to see."

Winston Churchill

The profession of nursing is experiencing rapid and dramatic change. Nurses in all settings are affected by these changes. This chapter analyzes the shift from acute to community-based care and its effect on nursing practice. Managed care and health care reform are discussed as factors contributing to the shift from acute to community-based care. Continuous quality improvement is presented as a means of maintaining high-quality care in a time of shrinking resources.

REVIEW

 I. Historical perspective of health care in the United States
    A. Legislation
       1. Entitlement programs
       2. Insurance
    B. Organization
       1. Governing bodies
    C. Environment of care
       1. Settings for the provision of health care
          a) Home
          b) Hospital
          c) Community

II. Health care policy and planning
   A. Legislative process
   B. Nurses' roles
      1. Organizations
      2. Political action
III. Economics of health care
   A. Cost of health care
   B. Payers of health care
      1. Consumers
      2. Employers
   C. Insurance companies
   D. Government
      1. Medicaid
         a) Insurance for low income people regardless of age
         b) Administered by state governments with federal control
      2. Medicare
         a) Federal health insurance for
            (1) People over 65
            (2) People under 65 with certain disabilities
      3. Types of insurance
         a) Fee for service
         b) HMO/PPO/DRG

DEFINITIONS

HMO: health maintenance organization

DRG: diagnosis-related group

PPO: preferred provider organization

Gatekeeper: a health care practitioner, such as a nurse or physician, who analyzes appropriateness of services such as specialty physician, laboratory, or radiology. The gatekeeper may work for a managed care program or for the coordinator of care, such as the primary care physician. The gatekeeper approves or denies requested services. In general, most of the gatekeeper's work is performed over the telephone. Clients are instructed as to where approved services must be obtained to receive coverage. The goal of the gatekeeper is cost containment through prevention of unnecessary services and utilization of the most cost-effective providers or services.

Capitation: "prepayment of a fixed periodic amount per patient. Each service is an expense charged against revenue" (Feldman & Kocin, 1991, p. 30). Insurance companies, both public and private, use actuarial data to determine average yearly cost of comprehensive medical care for a given population. This includes all primary, secondary, and tertiary health care services. Based on this information, the insurance company contracts with a provider or group to serve the designated population at a set (capitated) rate per person per month. The money is pooled by the provider or group and all health care costs for the population must be taken from that pool of money. If clients' service needs continue unchanged, statistically providers should see a predetermined profit. If unnecessary ancillary services are avoided, issues are resolved in ways other than office visits, and primary and preventive measures lead to a reduction in illnesses, providers will expend less of the "pot" of money. Often the remaining pool of money is distributed to the provider or group at the end of the year. This approach provides strong financial incentive to reduce preventable or unnecessary expenses.

Continuous quality improvement (CQI): "CQI involves a coordinated and integrated approach to improving processes that affect patient outcomes" (Sherman & Malkmus, 1994, p. 38).

DISCUSSION

Trends: Changes in the American Health Care System

WHY?

Economics, Access, and Quality.   The health care system in the United States is undergoing the most comprehensive transformation in its history. The traditional system of health care administration and utilization has led to uncontrolled costs in the public and private sectors. "Total health expenditures in the U.S. from all sources rose from $249.1 billion in 1980 to $604.1 billion in 1989" (Wassel, 1995, p. 24). If allowed to continue unchanged, Medicare funds will be depleted by the year 2002. Problems such as widespread fraud and abuse cost the Medicare system approximately 10% of its multibillion-dollar budget.

In a fee-for-service health care delivery system, there is little incentive for cost containment on the part of the provider or client. Providers' income depends on the number of office visits. Expensive specialty services may be sought out independently by clients, often without the benefit of expert guidance by a health care practitioner. Fee-for-service plans routinely pay for these and other costly services. Similarly, although preventive health care is viewed by providers as an important component of health care, there is financial disincentive to prevent illness in a fee-for-service model. The sicker the client, the more services required and the greater the revenue collected. Health care practitioners and public and private insurance programs have realized the cost of this approach, both financially and in terms of clients' health outcomes, and have called for reform of the system.

As the cost and percentage of gross national expenditure on health care continue to rise, the population of uninsured individuals is also growing. "Over 35 million Americans have no health care coverage, although two thirds of these individuals are either employed or the dependent of someone who is employed" (Bednash, 1994, p. 83). This has led to the provision of increasingly expensive health care to a diminishing percentage of the population. Clearly, the country's economic structure will not survive if this trend continues. To address these issues, health care must become both more accessible and more affordable.

HOW?

Health Care Reform.   Managed care is the country's response to problems in the health care delivery system. Because the definition of managed care varies, several examples are presented here.

"The term 'managed care' is used generically and encompasses a wide variety of health care programs and organizational structures that control or influence the access, costs and utilization of services within a select provider network" (Coleman, 1993, p. 2).

In the provision of health services through a single point of entry, the focus is on the provision of primary care with primary care providers controlling access to specialty physicians and other services. Clients are enrolled in plans in which the primary care provider may be determined for them. Patient care is managed to ensure an emphasis on quality, prevention, and primary care with the ultimate goal of reduction in inappropriate use of resources.

Prepayment arrangements, capitation, negotiated fees and discounts, and policies regarding prior authorization and quality assurance are part of managed care. Managed care programs have been in existence for decades in the form of HMOs, PPOs, DRGs, and various governmental insurance programs. These programs have demonstrated the ability to regulate the provision of quality care, at a reasonable cost, to a large population. Although there is much to learn about the expansion of these programs to the majority of the nation's populace, the recent crisis in health care has shed new light on the potential benefits of managed care systems. It is estimated that "80% of the nation's insured population will be enrolled in HMOs and PPOs before the turn of the century" (Coleman, 1993, p. 1).

In addition to renewed interest in managed care systems, there has been a trend toward partnerships between public and private insurance programs. This is seen in the increasing number of managed care systems operated by local and county entities. Government and private insurance companies are working together to identify mutual goals and areas of expertise with the aim of forming partnerships based on appropriate use of limited resources.

Managed care addresses the issues of quality improvement, cost containment, and increased access to health care in the following ways:

1. Reduction in inappropriate use of services through the use of gatekeepers
2. Capitation
3. Case management services
4. Provision of care in the community
5. Partnerships between public and private insurance providers
6. Continuous quality improvement

Continuous Quality Improvement. The intention of CQI is to "lower costs, increase revenue, enhance operations, improve clinical outcomes, prove service value, and create organization synergy" (Carefoote, 1994, p. 31). CQI, or total quality management (TQM), as it is often referred to, is accomplished through education and empowerment of employees to make changes that will lead to high-quality client care. The focus on improved outcomes along with lower costs has made CQI an important component of health care reform.

Most definitions of CQI are within the context of nurses' influence on individual patients or clients. Although this approach is well suited to the acute care environment, in certain areas of community health nursing the principles must be modified. Rather than focusing on individual client outcomes, community health nurses are responsible for promoting the health of aggregates and communities. This focus presents difficulties in the application of generalized CQI principles, which are geared to the clinical outcome and satisfaction of individual clients. Community health nurses must identify ways to modify CQI principles to assess outcome criteria for groups of clients.

WHERE?

The Community. "Early in the development of nursing, people were cared for in their home; hospitals developed not as meccas of scientific knowledge, but as society's response to the homeless and poor" (Liaschenko, 1994, p. 16). As the quote from Winston Churchill at the beginning of this chapter implies, history tends to repeat itself. We are entering an era in which the vast majority of health care services will be provided in the home (Clarke & Cody, 1994, p. 10). This shift is a result of many influencing factors, most notably the economics of health care. Simply put, it is usually less expensive to provide medical care for clients in their homes.

Potential benefits of the provision of health care in the community include:

Improved outcomes
> Research by nurses and other health care professionals has demonstrated the fact that the environment of care influences clients' responses to interventions. Most individuals prefer the milieu of the home to that of the hospital and consequentially experience better outcomes when care is provided in the home.

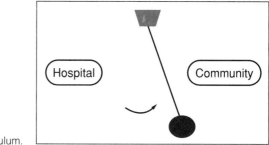

The pendulum.

Cost savings

> In many instances, the cost of hospitalization exceeds that of the provision of similar services in the home.

Cost shifting

> Appropriate community agencies will provide ancillary services, often at low or no cost to the client. Families become more involved with the care of the client when that care is provided in the home.

Client preference

Holistic approach to care

Ability to provide highly technical services in the home

Although the pendulum is swinging in the direction of community-based care, it is imperative that decisions about appropriate settings for health care be based on research related to outcomes. The home environment is not always the most appropriate place for care.

An example of an instance in which the shift toward community-based care may have been precipitous is that of early postpartum discharge. Many insurance companies, primarily managed care programs, viewed early discharge as a mutually beneficial endeavor. New mothers seemed to want to return home as soon as possible after delivery. Shorter hospital stays were appealing to insurance companies who experienced cost savings. Unfortunately, several factors were not considered:

- Initially clients were allowed the option of early discharge. Eventually, however, some insurance companies developed protocols requiring mothers and their babies to leave the hospital, in some circumstances as soon as 6 to 12 hours after delivery.
- The determination for eligibility for early discharge was often based solely on the medical condition of the mother and baby, without consideration of significant psychosocial factors.
- Many mothers and infants were returning to homes with inadequate support systems. This led to home environments placing the mothers at high risk for fatigue, depression, and stress, thus creating a situation ripe for problems such as postpartum depression and child abuse.
- Learning capacity was limited. Although they may have received education in the hospital, this education occurred at a highly stressful time with little opportunity for reinforcement.
- Clients were often unclear about warning signs, health indicators for mother and baby, and appropriate follow-up measures.

In this example, some early discharge clients experienced serious health consequences related to inappropriate follow-up care. This reinforces the fact that payers and providers must look at the appropriateness of alternative programs and ensure that the health care needs of clients are not overshadowed by the potential economic benefits. Insurance companies are now looking at nursing research related to improved outcomes when early discharge is accompanied by a postpartum home visit from a highly skilled nurse. It appears that cost savings and improved outcomes may be attained when early discharge programs are accompanied by appropriate follow-up in the home.

The success of managed care systems is contingent on the use of cost-effective professionals who are skilled in the provision of preventive and primary health care services in the home environment. Beginning with Florence Nightingale, nurses have been leaders in the area of community-based health care. Nurses have historically been advocates for the right of clients to receive care in the home. Nursing research focused on outcomes has demonstrated the efficacy of home-based care. This, along with ongoing research, will secure nursing's position as an integral part of successful reform of the health care delivery system.

Case Studies and Exercises

Responses to the following case studies and exercises reflect the ability to:

1. Consider personal attitudes and beliefs regarding preparedness for the future of nursing.
2. Acknowledge ongoing and imminent changes in the health care system of the United States.
3. Identify specific community health nursing roles and responsibilities in a managed care environment.
4. Analyze effects of health care reform on particular clients (individuals, families, and communities).
5. Apply the principles of CQI to particular scenarios.

2.1 EXERCISE

SELF-ANALYSIS

Questions

1) Why did you become/are you becoming a nurse?

2) How do you feel about the future of nursing? Discuss your response.

3) How have/will you prepare yourself for changes in health care?

2.2 E X E R C I S E

CULTURAL RELEVANCE

Review the information presented below and respond to the questions by discussing ways that you, as a community health nurse working for a community clinic, might address some of the consequences of health care reform.

Questions

Many managed care programs offer coverage for traditional health care services only. As a community health nurse, you realize that these services are not appropriate for a section of your client population that practices alternative medicine.

1) Will you work to ensure the option of alternative medicine coverage, through the managed care system, for your clients?
   - If so, how?

   - If not, defend your response.

2) Who will you involve in your approach?

3) What rationale will you use for your argument?

4) What, specifically, will you request from the managed care system?

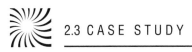 2.3 CASE STUDY

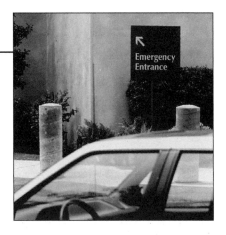

PROVIDER RELATIONS

SCENARIO

Provider Relations

Many providers have expressed dis-
satisfaction with the reimbursement
rates offered by the local managed
care system. Some providers have
begun to assign office visits for non-
emergency situations for 6 to 8 weeks
from the date of request, with the expectation that most clients will find an
alternative to the office visit. These providers blame low rates of capitation
on the inability to hire sufficient staff to accommodate all requested visits.
Some of these clients ultimately seek care in the emergency room. These
visits are charged against the provider's capitation amount, which has led
to even higher levels of frustration on the part of providers.

In this scenario, both providers and clients are becoming frustrated. As
a nurse in the managed care system, your duties include provider relations.
The capitated rate for providers is set by the state; it is not a negotiable
issue. The resources available to you include your time (20 h/wk) and the
assistance of a part-time health educator employed by the managed care
program.

Questions

1) What are your responsibilities to the clients of the managed care system?

2) What additional information do you need to address this issue?

3) How will you gather this information?

4) What do you perceive as the primary needs of the clients in this situation?

5) What do you perceive as the primary needs of providers in this situation?

6) What information will you provide in your educational outreach to:
   - Clients

   - Providers

   - Managed Care Organization

7) How will you determine the success of your outreach efforts?

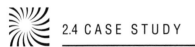 2.4 CASE STUDY

EARLY POSTPARTUM DISCHARGE

This chapter addressed an example of the effects of early postpartum discharge programs. This approach was seen as a way of reducing health care costs while increasing client satisfaction. When problems were identified in the early postpartum discharge programs, many agencies abandoned the concept immediately and reverted to previous standard lengths of stay.

SCENARIO

As a nurse working as the liaison between Capitol City Hospital and its home health agency, you are given the job of reviewing your early postpartum discharge program. Your program has been in effect for 18 months. Client satisfaction is high. The program has increased revenue for the hospital since many clients choose to deliver at Capitol City Hospital because of the early discharge program.

The protocol for your early discharge program includes a postpartum home visit by an RN from the home health agency. These visits are provided as a service to the client. In some cases visits are billable to insurance companies; Medicaid authorizes payment for one postpartum visit.

You have gathered the following information about the early discharge program:

1. Protocol: standard is one visit within 48 hours after discharge, which includes:

   Education

   > Newborn care
   > Breast-feeding
   > Warning signs warranting follow-up (mother and baby)
   >> Infection
   >> Hemorrhage
   > Comfort
   > Parenting
   > Sexuality
   >> Resumption of sexual activity
   >> Contraception
   > Community resources
   > Nutrition
   > Well and sick baby care

   Assessment

   > Infant: jaundice (heel stick performed if necessary)
   > Mother: hemorrhage, perineal lacerations, hematomas
   > Both
   >> Nutrition
   >> Weight
   >> Hydration
   >> Breast-feeding
   > Elimination

2. Cost

   - Fully reimbursed by some insurance companies
   - All mother-baby dyads receive postpartum visits, regardless of insurance coverage.
   - Optional or additional methods of reimbursement have not been explored by the agency.

- Agency makes money on reimbursed visits, loses money on non-reimbursed, but additional revenue generated by clients choosing the hospital because of the positive public perception program is thought to balance out cost of nonreimbursed visits.

3. Outcomes: outcomes of postpartum early discharge with accompanying home visit (as compared with traditional length of postpartum stay)

   Positive

   - Higher percentage of successful (at least 2 months) breast-feeding
   - Higher rate of immunization compliance
   - Fewer inappropriate emergency room visits
   - High client satisfaction
   - Lower levels of maternal stress reported to pediatricians

   Negative

   - Higher incidence in jaundice in babies whose mothers participated in the early discharge program

Questions

1) What, if any, additional information do you need to make a recommendation regarding the program?

   - How will you obtain this information?

2) As the nurse making a recommendation for the continuation or termination of the postpartum early discharge program, what are your recommendations?
   - Should the program be abandoned?

   - Should the program be maintained?

3) What, if any, alterations would you make in the following areas:
   - Funding

   - Protocol
         Client education

         Assessment

         Timing of Visit

4) Outcome measurements are critical to demonstrate the efficacy of this program.
   - What will you evaluate?

   - How often?

   - Why?

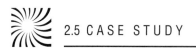 2.5 CASE STUDY

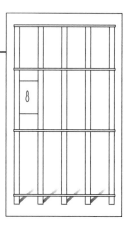

CLINICAL SERVICES

SCENARIO

You are a nurse working in the prison in Metropolis. You oversee clinic operations. You have been receiving complaints from both providers and clients (inmates) regarding the flow in the prison tuberculosis (TB) clinic. Clients complain that they are waiting too long to receive services. They claim that clinic times coincide with outdoor activity/smoking time and are angry about being denied this "right." Additionally, providers in the clinic are concerned about perceived inefficient use of their time. Examples include long periods of "down time" with no clients to be seen, followed by several high acuity clients presenting at the same time.

The TB clinic is held twice each month. Providers, both physicians and nurse practitioners, come from the local health department to staff the clinic. Their time is limited to 3 hours per clinic. Usually one physician and one nurse practitioner staff each clinic. Responsibilities of these providers include examination of radiographs, review of medication administration and compliance, review of laboratory results including sputum specimens, and recommendations for follow-up measures including medication, laboratory, and x-ray, and isolation as necessary.

The number of clients on an average clinic day ranges from 10 to 25, with varying degrees of acuity. The current process for the TB clinic is as follows:

- Inmates (clients) are scheduled for clinic.
  - All clients warranting services are scheduled for clinic visits are scheduled every 15 minutes, to accommodate safety needs of guards bringing inmates to and from the clinic.
  - Some visits take 3 minutes, others may last up to 25 minutes.
- Clients are seen by the first available provider.
  - Occasionally the nurse practitioner will see a client who, for evaluation purposes, must then be seen by the physician.
  - Clients are to be counseled by prison nursing staff, both before being seen by the provider and after the examination.
- Prior to the visit
  - Nursing staff review medication compliance and assess for complications.
- After the visit
  - Nursing staff review the results of the examination and arrange for necessary follow-up procedures.

Questions

Using the principles of CQI, respond to the following questions.

1) What are the actual and potential problems in this scenario as they affect:

   ● Providers

   ● Clients

   ● Prison staff

2) What are the variables that you, as clinic coordinator, have to work with?

3) What are the goals of your actions related to this scenario?

4) What interventions will you make to achieve these goals?

2.6 EXERCISE

TRENDS IN NURSING ROLES

Questions

How do you think the following factors will influence the future of nursing?

1) Cost containment

2) Limited resources

3) The "graying" (aging) of the American population

4) More nursing care being provided in the community setting

5) Increasing need for nurses to document and research to justify the impact of their work

References

Bednash, G. (1994). The future of nursing and health care reform. Keynote speech 4/20/94. National Student Nurses Association. *NSNA/Imprint,* September/October, 83–85.

Carefoote, R. (1994). Total quality management implementation in home care agencies. *Journal of Nursing Administration, 24*(10), 31–37.

Clarke, P., & Cody, W. (1994). Nursing theory–based practice in the home and community: The crux of professional nursing education. *Advancements in Nursing Science, 17*(2), 41–53.

Coleman, J. (1993). Medical case management and managed care. *The Case Manager, 4*(1), 39–45.

Feldman, R., & Kocin, M. (1991). Caring for disoriented clients with Alzheimer's disease at home. *Journal of Home Health Care Practice, 3*(4), 40–47.

Liaschenko, J. (1994). The moral geography of home care. *Advancements in Nursing Science, 17*(2), 16–26.

Sherman, J., & Malkmus, M. (1994). Integrating quality assurance and total quality management/quality improvement. *Journal of Nursing Administration, 24*(3), 37–41.

Wassel, M. (1995). Occupation health nursing and the advent of managed care. *American Association of Occupational Health Nurses Journal, 43*(1), 23–28.

CHAPTER 3

Community Health Nursing in the 21st Century

"Never before have we had so little time in which to do so much."

Franklin D. Roosevelt

The trend toward the provision of health care outside the hospital setting has led to changes in employment opportunities and educational requirements for nurses. Projections regarding nursing employment indicate that the majority of nurses will soon be practicing in the community setting. Chapter 3 presents statistical information regarding this trend and identifies the potential impact on nurses, both individually and collectively.

REVIEW

I. Nursing employment statistics
    A. Acute
        1. Hospital based
    B. Nonacute
        1. Community based
    C. Entry to practice
II. Nursing education
    A. Types of programs
        1. BSN
        2. ADN
        3. Diploma

DISCUSSION _____

Statistical Overview of Trends in Nursing Employment

Currently there are over 2.2 million nurses in the United States, 83% of whom are actively employed (U.S. Department of Health and Human Services [USDHHS], 1994). Two thirds of nurses are working in the hospital setting at a time when 40% of hospital beds are empty. Clearly, managed care is leading to a diminishing hospital-based client sector.

As the number of clients cared for in the hospital decreases, the acuity level of hospital patients is increasing. As hospitals focus increasingly on intensive care and outpatient services, nurses working in the acute care setting will be required to have a high level of technical skill and must be cross-trained to cover a variety of nursing specialty areas. Many nurses will be leaving the hospital for community-based nursing practice. Estimates indicate health care reform can create 600,000 to 700,000 new opportunities for nurses (Ketter, 1994, p. 23). These nurses, moving from the acute to the community setting, will focus on primary and preventive care services as well as technical nursing care in the home.

Most experts agree that within 5 years, less than half of all nurses will be employed in hospitals. This shift requires changes in the composition of the basic nursing work force. It is incumbent on nurses to clarify the roles of the Bachelor of Science in Nursing (BSN) and the Associate Degree in Nursing (ADN) in the field of community health nursing. Matching educational preparation with appropriate job duties will likely lead to an era in which bachelor's and master's prepared nurses function in an autonomous role and associate degree nurses provide technical care to clients in their homes. Regardless of the evolution of these roles, it is critical to the profession of nursing that all nurses have the skills and knowledge base necessary for effective community health nursing practice.

EDUCATION

As Figure 3-1 illustrates, the nursing profession is experiencing a period of rapid change. The shift from acute to community-based nursing practice is imminent. Consideration must be given to educational requirements for entry level community-based nursing practice.

The genesis of health care reform has spurred renewed interest in the discussion of entry to professional nursing practice. The BSN degree has long been considered the minimum requirement for entry to community-based nursing practice. Exceptions have been made in certain situations, but the consensus of the nursing profession has been that the education offered in a BSN program is necessary for preparation of a professional community health nurse.

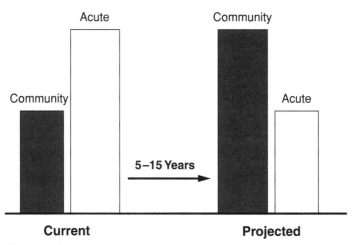

FIGURE 3-1   Trends in nursing employment.

Associate degree programs have historically emphasized preparation of nurses to meet the technical needs of patients in the acute care setting. Increasingly, these programs are focusing on the development of critical thinking skills as applied to the community setting. BSN programs will continue to provide a strong theoretical base as well as focusing on the development of independent professional judgment in preparation for autonomous nursing practice.

All nurses, regardless of their educational preparation, must assess their readiness to practice nursing in the 21st century. Increasing knowledge about current and future opportunities will assist nurses in the analysis of relevance and adequacy of their education and professional nursing experience.

To address the demand for professional nurses, schools and departments of nursing have a responsibility to offer ADN-prepared nurses opportunities to work toward their BSN. Universities must offer ADN to BSN programs that are accessible and affordable. Ideally, these "bridge" programs should be offered at various times and in convenient locations to accommodate the schedules of nurses, many of whom are working full-time.

"The Department of Health and Human Services estimates that by the year 2000 there will be half as many baccalaureate and higher degree nurses as are needed, and an oversupply of nearly 20% of associate degree nurses" (USDHSS, 1991). This discrepancy presents both opportunity and challenge to nursing. Analyzing and codifying the roles of the various levels of nurses in the community setting will reduce frustration and unrealistic expectations on the part of the employer, client, and nurse. Additionally, this proactive approach will reduce dissent within the nursing profession.

TRAINING AND SKILLS

Although preparation for community nursing practice requires the acquisition or update of skills and theory base, many skills are universally applicable in nursing practice. Presented below are cognitive and psychomotor skills from acute care nursing practice that are transferable to the community setting. Subsequent chapters will present additional skills and knowledge base required for effective nursing practice in the community setting.

Transferable skills include:

- Historical and physical assessment
- Patient advocacy
- Quality assurance
- Utilization review
- Technical expertise
- Medication administration
- Communication skills
- Triage/prioritization skills
- Computer skills
- Knowledge and application of nurse practice standards

Comparison of Acute and Community Nursing Practice

Community health nursing is the practice of nursing in the "environment of care," such as homes, schools, and other sites in the community. Table 3-1

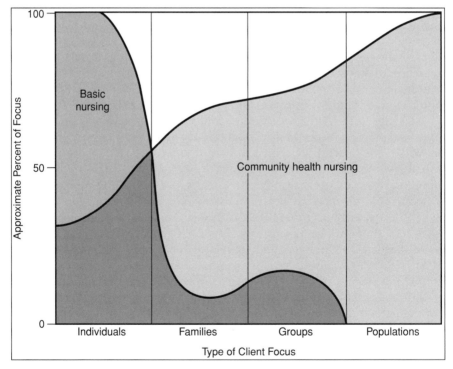

Client focus in community-based nursing practice. From Spradley and Allender (1996), with permission.

TABLE 3-1
Comparison of Metaparadigm Concepts in Hospital Setting and Home Setting

Metaparadigm Concept	Hospital Setting	Home Setting
Human being	Less than 1% of the population. A "patient": an individual usually separated from family and often typologized by disease entity (eg, "cancer patient").	Over 95% of the population; person and family as client; group or community as client; personal and cultural identity easily seen.
Environment	Standardized room, ward, or specialized unit; a work setting for health care professionals, with access severely limited for most others (like family, friends). The place and manner in which the person lives remain mostly unknown.	Natural, sociocultural, and symbolic environments shared with family and community in dynamic interchange with the human being. The client and environment cannot be separated and are not mutually exclusive.
Health	Dichotomized with illness; considered its polar opposite and as such the goal of care; when health is objectively appraised as "good," person is ejected.	Includes illness as an aspect of life; goal of care is most often viewed as the quality of life experienced by the person, family, or community.
Nursing	Activities largely delegated by physicians; centered on treatment of illness through medication, technology; short-term, predictable interventions; majority of current practices require no more than a 2-year degree.	Largely autonomous practice; interventions tend to be mutually negotiated with clients based on client values and require broad knowledge on nurse's part; nurse–client interactions and goals are longer term, oriented toward quality of life; baccalaureate education required for effective practice.

From Clarke and Cody (1994), with permission.

contains distinctions of metaparadigm concepts between acute and community-based nursing practice.

Case Studies and Exercises

Responses to the following case studies and exercises reflect the ability to:

1. Outline opportunities for professional development.
2. Analyze employment options.
3. Consider personal preparedness for community-based nursing practice.
4. Compare and contrast skills used in acute and community settings.
5. Match nurses' skills with available employment opportunities.

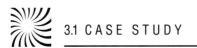 3.1 CASE STUDY

EMPLOYMENT OPTIONS

SCENARIO

You are a nurse working in the car-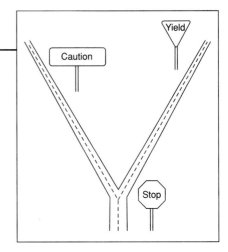
diac intensive care unit (CICU) in
Capitol City Hospital. Your hospital
has recently been purchased by a
health maintenance organization
(HMO). Rumors about downsizing of
nursing staff are rampant among hospital employees. Realizing that many
nurses have more seniority than you
do, you decide to make an appointment with your supervisor to discuss the
rumors and assess your status with the hospital. Your supervisor advises
you that layoffs are indeed imminent and that given your date of hire there
is a high likelihood that you are at risk of "termination."

Your situation is as follows. You received an ADN 10 years ago. You
worked as an RN on the medical-surgical unit for 6 years at Capitol City
Hospital. Four years ago you left your permanent position to work part-
time on the evening shift to continue your education and receive a BSN.
Your goal in returning to school was to prepare yourself for either a super-
visory position in the hospital or future practice in the community setting.
You completed your BSN 2 years ago and subsequently obtained your permanent position in the CICU.

During your BSN education, you precepted with one of the local managed care program administrators and became interested in managed care.
Your county has operated a managed care program for 2 years. Your preceptor encouraged you to apply for a position as a nurse liaison, but you
decided to return to work at Capitol City Hospital because you felt that you
lacked the experience necessary for a position in the community setting.

Recently, you were approached by a neighbor who volunteers for his
daughter's school. He informed you of a vacancy in the position of school
nurse. This position was appealing to you because of the proximity to your
home as well as the flexible schedule. Once again, however, you gave it little serious consideration due to your perceived lack of experience.

Glancing in the classified section of the newspaper last Sunday, you
noticed advertisements for the following nursing positions:

- Clinic nurse in the local health department
- Occupational health nurse for a computer company in Metropolis

You now have four possible community health nursing employment
avenues to pursue:

- Managed care
- School nursing
- Clinic nurse
- Occupational health nurse

Questions

1) List factors that must be considered when analyzing employment opportunities:

  - Salary

  - Job location

  - Flexibility in hours

  - Professional challenge

  - Opportunity for advancement

  - Personal comfort level with existing skills (versus challenge of learning new job)

  - Adequacy of personal skills and knowledge base

2) Given the scenario, list all actual and potential options:

  - Continue in present position and hope that position is not eliminated

  - Analyze options for advancement within Capitol City Hospital

  - Identify means of securing current position

  - Contact your preceptor to explore employment opportunities with a managed care program

  - Apply for community health nurse position
    - School nurse
    - Occupational health nurse
    - Clinic nurse

After careful consideration, you decide to apply for the school nursing position. Although the salary is lower than that of other positions, the flexible hours and convenient location are appealing to you. Additionally, you feel that you have sufficient skills and that this position will prepare you for future opportunities in community health nursing.

You apply for the position in May. You are offered the position, which will begin in August, with the stipulation that you increase your knowledge of the principles and practices of school nursing. You will remain in your current position over the summer.

3) How will you prepare yourself, over the next 3 months, for your new role as school nurse?

  - Literature reviews
    - Community health nursing texts
    - Journals

- Peer support
  - Connect with local school nurses
  - Join community health nursing organization

- Clarify expectations

- Identify "clients"

- Coursework
  - Continuing education
  - Community health nursing updates

- Licensure/education

3.2 EXERCISE

PROFESSIONAL DEVELOPMENT OPPORTUNITIES

Discuss opportunities available in your community for the following areas of professional nursing development. How would you go about obtaining additional information about these opportunities?

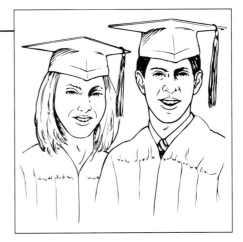

Opportunities	Time (hours offered)	Location	Cost	Prerequisites
RN to BSN				
BSN to MSN				
Advanced Practice (ie, Nurse Practitioner)				
MPH (Masters in Public Health)				

(continued)

Opportunities	Time (hours offered)	Location	Cost	Prerequisites
Doctorate Programs DNS (Doctorate in Nursing Science)				
EDD (Educational Doctorate)				
Other:				

3.3 EXERCISE

NURSING EMPLOYMENT OPTIONS

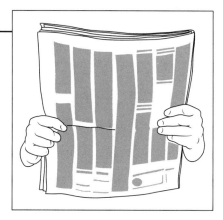

Look through the classified section of at least two newspapers serving your community.

Questions

1) What types of nursing positions are available in your community?

2) Do you find the type of nursing position you envision for your future represented in your search?

3) What other, more effective means might you use to identify employment opportunities in your desired area of practice?

4) Are there geographic differences in opportunities for your desired area of practice?

5) What skills and experience will convince employers to hire you as the best candidate for your desired position?

6) How will you obtain information about employers' expectations for the ideal candidate for this position?

7) What, if any, additional preparation, educational or experiential, will make you a stronger candidate for your desired position?

3.4 EXERCISE

REPARATION FOR COMMUNITY HEALTH NURSING PRACTICE

Questions

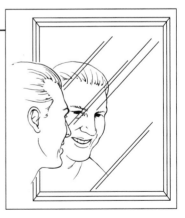

1) Identify three areas in which you must increase your knowledge or skills to better prepare yourself for the practice of community health nursing.

2) In your opinion, what responsibilities do the following entities have to provide opportunities for professional nursing development?
   ● Professional nursing organizations

   ● Nursing education

   ● Employers of nurses

3) What additional opportunities do you feel would benefit the nurses in your community?

3.5 EXERCISE

COMPARISON OF ACTIVITIES

Effective nursing practice in the community requires creativity, flexibility, and resourcefulness. Given the following situations, state ways in which the performance of nursing interventions may vary when comparing the acute and the community setting.

Questions

1) Washing hands and donning gloves before inserting a Foley catheter
   ● Acute care setting: cardiac ICU

   ● Community setting: small, overcrowded apartment with one communal bathroom

2) Follow-up per client's complaint of chest pain and shortness of breath
   - Acute care setting: hospital's orthopedic rehabilitation unit

   - Community setting: prison

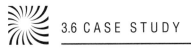 3.6 CASE STUDY

TRANSITIONING AND EXPECTATIONS

SCENARIO

George worked as an RN in the recovery room of Brownsville Hospital for 23 years. Recently, his son and daughter-in-law had their first child. George decided to move from Brownsville to Capitol City to be near his new grandchild. In seeking employment opportunities, George realized that his options were limited. During his years with Brownsville Hospital, George had taken general nursing review courses and some continuing education courses in gerontology.

By reviewing positions that would call on his skills and meet his salary requirements, George decided to apply for the following positions:
- Evening shift charge nurse in the Capitol City jail
- Clinic nurse for a local community clinic
- Entry level home health nurse specializing in gerontology

George was offered, and accepted, the home health nursing position. He was pleased with the training offered to him as a part of his orientation process. He was particularly appreciative of the comprehensive review of gerontology. Feeling confident with his knowledge of gerontology, as well as his mastery of the agency's complex forms, George was ready to make his first home visit.

George would observe one home visit before performing independent visits. George's first visit was with Mary Ann, an experienced home health nurse. George and Mary Ann's client was Harlan, an 82-year-old man with cirrhosis of the liver and esophageal varices.

Although George felt comfortable performing technical skills related to Harlan's care, he experienced extreme anxiety when attempting to communicate with Harlan. George could not understand why he was having difficulty interacting with his client; he had been a nurse for over 25 years, he was considered one of the best nurses in his unit, and here he was feeling completely inept. George was amazed at the ease with which Mary Ann solicited assessment data from the client. She asked questions about Harlan's family, his disease process, even his alcoholism. George felt that he could never communicate with clients in such a manner.

That evening George gave careful consideration to his ability to function effectively as a home health nurse. He could not come to terms with the difference in competence that he felt in the community, as opposed to the acute care setting. George decided to request a reassignment from his supervisor to avoid the discomfort that he experienced with the home visit.

Questions

1) Is George incompetent? Discuss your reaction to George's expectations of his performance.

2) How might the following novice home health nurse's reaction have been different:

  • A 25-year-old newly graduated BSN with no previous health care experience

  • A hospice nurse who recently completed and ADN to BSN program

  • A new graduate who volunteered for the Senior Citizen Home Nutrition Program while in nursing school

3) What additional education and or assistance does George need to continue in his position?

4) How might he go about obtaining the necessary skills for effective community health nursing practice?

References

Clarke, P., & Cody, W. (1994). Nursing theory–based practice in the home and community: The crux of professional nursing education. *Advances in Nursing Science, 17*(2), 41–53.

Ketter, J. (1994, October). Finding opportunity in change. *The American Nurse,* 21–23.

Spradley, B. W., & Allender, J. A. (1996). *Community health nursing concepts and practice* (4th ed.). Philadelphia, PA: Lippincott-Raven Publishers.

United States Department of Health and Human Services. (1991). *Health personnel in the United States: Seventh report to Congress, 1990.* Washington, DC: US Government Printing Office.

United States Department of Health and Human Services. (1994). *The registered nurse population 1992: Findings from the National Sample Survey of Registered Nurses.* Washington, DC: US Government Printing Office.

PART
II

KEY CONCEPTS

CHAPTER 4

Application of the Nursing Process in the Environment of Care

"In the absence of clearly defined goals, we are forced to concentrate on activity and ultimately become enslaved by it."

Chuck Coonradt

Understanding the application of the nursing process with clients in the community is critical for effective nursing practice in this setting. Chapter 4 provides a review of the components of the nursing process. The discussion highlights considerations of the application of this process in the environment of care. Nurses who are well versed in the principles of the nursing process, and are able to apply those principles in the community setting, are equipped to address the multitude of issues they will encounter in the community setting.

REVIEW

The nursing process is the cornerstone of professional nursing practice. It is this fundamental process that links all nurses, regardless of practice setting. The application of the nursing process with all clients ensures interactions that are focused on identified goals. This chapter provides an overview of the nursing process and addresses specific considerations of its application in the community as the environment of care.

The nursing process is referenced throughout this text as a means of approaching cases. Although there are variations in terminology related to the process, the following steps are used in this text:

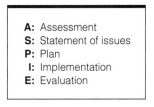

> **A:** Assessment
> **S:** Statement of issues
> **P:** Plan
> **I:** Implementation
> **E:** Evaluation

I. Assessment

This is the stage of information gathering. Nurses make assessments based on subjective and objective information. Any information that may affect the client should be considered as potentially relevant assessment data. Information is obtained through physical, environmental, and psychosocial assessments; laboratory and x-ray findings; and nursing history.

II. Problem statement

In this step the nurse presents a nursing diagnosis that includes possible etiologies of identified problems.

III. Plan

Based on the previous two steps, the nurse develops a plan of action specific to the needs of the client. The nurse must work in conjunction with the client to determine the course of action as well as the desired outcome or goal.

IV. Implementation

Nursing interventions include treatments, education, and data gathering, which are directed toward achievement of identified goals.

V. Evaluation

Evaluation involves an examination of the effectiveness of nursing actions and identification of the degree to which goals have been attained.

DISCUSSION

Considerations in the Environment of Care

ASSESSMENT

In the acute care setting it is often difficult for nurses to obtain detailed information about clients' families and communities. Working in the community, however, nurses may be overwhelmed with such information. Objective information about clients' families, aggregates, and communities is presented to nurses when they enter the environment of care. Nurses must develop skills in acquiring subjective and specific objective information that will provide relevant assessment data.

Active listening is an important tool for all nurses. Nurses working in the community gather relevant subjective data from clients as well as families, friends, and others who may be present in the environment of care.

Nurses working in the community use many of the assessment tools used in the acute care setting. Physical assessment and examination of laboratory and x-ray results are common examples.

Subjective and objective data are gathered using the following techniques:

- Needs assessment of individual, family, aggregate, and community
- Assessment of strengths of individual, family, aggregate, and community
- Assessment of home environment
- Active listening
- Observation of interpersonal interactions

Assessment Tools.   Tools and techniques that may assist the nurse in performing a comprehensive assessment in the community setting include:

- Individual assessment
  - Medical history
  - Patient history forms
  - Nutritional status
        Diet recall forms
        Prescriptions for feedings, supplements, diet
  - Growth charts
  - Emotional, intellectual, and developmental assessments tools
  - Physical and motor development assessment tools
  - Benefits available through insurance
- Family assessment
  - Identification of family composition
  - Review of family resources
  - Discussion of family's decision-making process
  - Caretaker or support system
- Home assessment
  - Home safety assessment tools
  - Analysis of space issues such as number of individuals in home
  - Number of rooms, levels of home, age of home
- Community assessment
  - Observation of client locale in relation to community services
  - Information may be obtained by:
        Drive-through "windshield survey"
        Chamber of Commerce
        Local media

STATEMENT OF ISSUES

Historically, nurses' efforts have focused on the identification of 'weaknesses' and resolution of clients' problems. An example of this is the nursing diagnosis. Although the nursing diagnosis remains a valuable tool, the focus on clients' problems has been altered in recent years and more emphasis is being placed on the significance of clients' strengths. This approach is well suited to the practice of nursing in the community because it identifies potential resources to be used in the planning stage of the nursing process.

In this phase of the nursing process, assessment data are used to identify clients' problems, potential problems, and strengths. Using assessment data to identify strengths and problems of the family, aggregate, and community is also necessary given their impact on the health of the client. Information relevant to this portion of the nursing process includes:

- Identified strengths of client, family, aggregate, and community
- Identified problems of client, family, aggregate, and community (ie, nursing diagnosis)
- Potential problems

PLAN

Planning for positive outcomes requires the client's involvement at each level of the nursing process. Planning the course of action requires intensive involvement of the client as well as others, such as family members, involved in the care of the client. This is particularly important in the community setting because the majority of follow-up is performed by the client and the family. Based on assessment data, nurses and clients work to develop realistic goals given the client's physiologic status as well as the psychosocial factors influencing the client, family and community.

Prioritizing Issues.   Planning for client care requires prioritization of identified actual and potential problems. In prioritizing, the nurse and client must address the following issues:

- Legal obligation to follow up (ie, reporting of abuse or neglect)
- Agency's goal (stated purpose of the visit)
- Client's goals (what client needs or values from the interaction with the community health nurse)

Ranking issues in order of importance to the nurse and client will begin the process of developing a mutual plan of action. Consideration of client strengths will assist in the development of a mutual approach to goal attainment that capitalizes on available resources, both internal and external. Prioritization of issues affecting the client is imperative for the development of a plan of action that is realistic and deals with the most critical of the client's needs. Planning for appropriate resource use requires consideration of the following:

- Availability of resource in the community
- Client's perception of resource

- Client's willingness and ability to use resource
- Logistics (ie, proximity of resource, hours of operation, etc)
- Cost
- Insurance coverage
- Options for payment

IMPLEMENTATION

Collaboration is the underlying theme in the implementation phase of the nursing process in the community setting. To increase the likelihood of accomplishing mutually identified goals, nurses must collaborate with the following individuals or groups:

- Identified client
- Family
- Aggregate
- Community
- Others involved in client's care
- Health care professionals
- Community resources

Common community health nurse interventions include:

- Physical assessment
- Performance of invasive and noninvasive procedures
- Education of client and family
- Ongoing information gathering
- Contracting with clients
- Referrals

EVALUATION

Evaluation is based on defined goals. The evaluation process must include the nurse, client, and additional support persons as desired by the client. This process will answer the following questions:

1. In what way were the objectives met?
2. What was not accomplished?
3. Do we need to revise the plan?
4. Is any further information necessary?
5. Are the family and community resources sufficient for achievement of this goal?

Case Studies and Exercises

Responses to the following case studies and exercises reflect the ability to:

1. Review complex, detailed cases and identify issues relevant for community health nurse intervention.
2. Compare and contrast nursing interventions given various nursing roles.

3. Analyze assessment data for relevance, significance, and degree of completeness.
4. Use available assessment data to identify clients' problems and strengths, both actual and potential.
5. Develop a plan for nursing intervention.
6. Prioritize issues based on client's situation and available resources.
7. Detail community health nursing implementation activities, including delegation of activities.
8. Identify outcome criteria for evaluating community health nursing intervention.

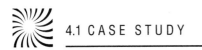 4.1 CASE STUDY

POSTPARTUM TEEN PARENTS

CASE INFORMATION

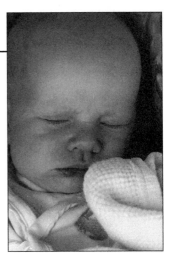

You are a home health nurse whose job duties include postpartum home visitation of clients after early discharge from the hospital. Your identified clients for this morning's visit are Jennifer and her newborn daughter Clare. You will be visiting this family twice, today for the 2-day postpartum visit and again a week from today.

Previsit Information: Demographics

CLIENTS

- Jennifer: 19 years old, primipara. She did not complete high school but recently passed the GED. Jennifer is employed as a waitress at a local restaurant. Her primary language is English.
- Clare: 2 days old.

FAMILY

Joe is Jennifer's husband. He is also 19 years old. Information on the medical record lists Joe's employment as auto mechanic and education as GED. His primary language is also English.

EXTENDED FAMILY

No information about the extended family is available before the visit.

COMMUNITY

The family lives in a mobile home park in Smithville. The home has one large and one small bedroom.

Purpose of Visit

IDENTIFIED PROBLEMS AND ISSUES

MEDICAL

Jennifer began receiving prenatal care in the first trimester of her pregnancy She missed five appointments because she had no transportation. Her identified medical problems during pregnancy included anemia and insufficient weight gain. Total weight gain for this pregnancy was 17 pounds. Jennifer's labor was 18 hours long and was uncomplicated. She suffered a third degree laceration during parturition.

PSYCHOSOCIAL

Given the limited information available from the medical record, the only identified psychosocial issues include lack of transportation and potential problems related to Jennifer and Jack's ages.

Statement of Problems, Issues, and Strengths

Before your visit to this family's home, you must plan your approach with the limited amount of information available to you. Begin your planning by identifying the following information as it relates to Jennifer, Clare, and the family system:

- Strengths
  - Acquisition of GED
  - Both Jennifer and Joe employed
  - Jennifer sought early prenatal care
- Actual problems
  - Altered nutrition: less than body requirements
  - Anemia
  - Lack of transportation
  - Third degree perineal laceration
- Potential problems
  - Risk for altered parenting related to parental age and inexperience
  - Risk for social isolation related to peer group response
  - Financial difficulties
  - Employment
  - Child care
  - Housing
  - Situational stress related to:
      Care of newborn
      Sleep deprivation
  - Risk for infection related to bacterial invasion subsequent to third degree perineal laceration
  - Altered nutrition
      Risk for ineffective breast feeding
      Risk for colonic constipation (Jennifer)
  - Risk for noncompliance with scheduled medical follow-up visits due to transportation problems

- ○ Knowledge deficit
    - Signs and symptoms warranting medical follow-up
- Identified needs
    - ○ Physical assessment of Jennifer
        - Laceration/perineum—hemorrhage, infection
        - Lochia
        - Fundus
        - Vital signs
        - Breast examination
    - ○ Physical assessment of Clare
        - Feeding patterns
        - Elimination
        - Nutritional status
        - Reflexes
        - Cord
        - Jaundice
        - Sleeping patterns and position
        - Vital signs
    - ○ Educational needs of postpartum primipara
        - Breast-feeding
        - Nutrition
        - Elimination
        - Self-examination of breast
        - Signs and symptoms warranting medical attention
        - Information about physical assessment results
    - ○ Educational needs of family unit
        - Parenting
        - Safety
            - Car seat
        - Cardiopulmonary resuscitation (CPR)
        - Management of therapeutic regime
        - Care of newborn
            - Appropriate clothing
        - Bathing
        - Thermoregulation and use of a thermometer
        - Family planning and resumption of sexual activity
    - ○ Psychosocial assessment of family unit
        - Bonding
        - Support for young family
        - Extended family
        - Peer support
        - Religious affiliation
        - Available resources
            - Housing
            - Financial
            - Employment

- ○ Child care
- ○ Parenting
  - Experience with newborns
  - Role models for parenting
- ○ Substance use or abuse

Previsit Plan

This is a case in which you will likely have a brief relationship with your clients. In planning for the visit with this young family you must be cognizant of the constraints of time and clients' attention during this period of major change in their lives. A reasonable period of time for this visit is 1½ to 2 hours. Given the number of real and actual problems in this situation, you must plan your visit by prioritizing the issues you can realistically address in two brief visits.

PREVISIT ACTIVITIES

Telephone prior to visit:

1. Introduce yourself and your role.
2. Discuss the purpose of the visit.
3. Set up or confirm appointment time.
4. Ask for directions.
5. Ask clients about information they would like you to bring on to the visit.
   - Collect and organize relevant educational and reference materials.
   - Gather necessary equipment: scale, thermometer, stethoscope, laboratory equipment for heel stick.

VISIT ACTIVITIES

The presumptive plan for today's visit, which may change according to assessment data gathered in the home, is as follows:

- Neighborhood assessment
- Establish rapport
- Identify parents' questions and concerns
- Obtain further data related to prioritized issues
  - ○ Support
  - ○ Nutrition
  - ○ Laceration
  - ○ Care of the newborn
- Physical assessment
- Education related to prioritized issues
- Anticipatory guidance
- Referral to area resources
- Plan next visit

Scenario

As you drive through the neighborhood you note the following significant information. The mobile home park is located on a road with a moderate amount of agricultural truck traffic, approximately 2 miles from downtown Smithville; there is a gas station and a small convenience store within three blocks of the home; within the mobile home park roads are well maintained; a small grassy area lies in the center of the park. The family's home is obviously old but has personalized touches such as a small garden and assorted potted plants. As you approach the entryway you notice several ashtrays, filled with cigarette butts, on the porch.

Jennifer answers the door and invites you into the home. You accept her invitation to sit on the couch in the front room. You observe that the house, although cluttered, appears to be clean. The front room is sparsely furnished and the lighting is dim. Joe is in the kitchen washing dishes. As you turn to sit down he dries his hands and leaves to another part of the home. Clare is sleeping in a car seat in the front room.

Nursing Process

ASSESSMENT

ESTABLISHING RAPPORT

Joe's departure from the front room affects your approach to the development of rapport. Although Jennifer and Clare are the identified clients, it is best to include all significant members of the family system to ensure a holistic approach to the nursing process.

NURSING ACTIONS

You ask Jennifer if Joe feels comfortable participating in the visit. She states that he thought the visit was "just for me and Clare." When Joe learns that he is a welcome participant he joins you in the front room.

1. Remind the couple that you are a nurse from the home health agency.
2. Review the purpose and expected length of the visit.
3. Advise the clients that the information shared during the visit is confidential and advise them of your legal responsibilities for reporting.
4. Advise them that the visit will involve both physical assessment and health education and that they will be asked to provide information that will help in providing appropriate care and education.
5. Ask them if they have any questions.
6. Ask them to discuss the labor and delivery experience.

PROBLEM-ORIENTED ASSESSMENT

SUPPORT

You discuss with the couple the fact that coming home from the hospital with a new baby can be difficult and ask open-ended questions about their experience. You ask them if they feel they have a supportive environment and ask specific questions about extended family, friends, and community or religious support networks.

Jennifer and Joe state that they feel "a little nervous" about the addition to the family, that they know they face major changes in their relationship. They say that although most of their friends are commuting to

Jonestown to attend junior college, they feel that the friends will continue to be supportive. Jennifer's mother lives in town and works full-time as a medical secretary. "She thought she was too young to be a grandmother at first, but now she just loves it," says Jennifer. Jennifer's mother plans on making dinner for the couple twice a week and will baby-sit as her schedule allows.

Joe's extended family members live in another state. His mother will be coming in a week to stay in the home and assist the couple. They are unsure about sleeping arrangements.

They state they have no affiliations with religious or community groups.

RESOURCES

You discuss with the couple the fact that you noted information related to their employment status on the medical record. You express the fact that having a child can lead to major changes in families' financial and employment situations. You ask them if they would like to discuss the impact Clare's birth will have on their financial status. You advise the couple that you do not need specific information about their financial status but you may be able to identify resources they might find helpful.

The couple seems uncomfortable discussing the topic of finances but they state that Jennifer will be staying home with Clare for the time being while Joe increases his hours at work. They add that the fact that they have only one vehicle has made it difficult for them to keep scheduled appointments. "We're trying to figure out how to get Clare and Jennifer to their doctor's appointments since I'll have the car and I work so far from home," says Joe.

NUTRITION

After advising the couple that you would like to discuss the nutritional problems experienced during pregnancy, as well as current nutritional status, Joe states "she was working too much back then . . . I told her to take better care of herself and to eat more . . . now that she'll be staying home with the baby everything should be fine." Jennifer states that she has continued to take her prenatal vitamins as instructed by her physician.

LACERATION

Jennifer states "the nurses told me some stuff about how to take care of the cut down there; I know I have to use this bottle with warm water to wash and that I have to be real careful but that's all I remember. I have an appointment to go back and see my doctor in about 2 weeks."

CARE OF THE NEWBORN

Joe and Jennifer state that they have had little experience with newborns. They have recently begun caring for a 4-year-old neighbor while her mother goes shopping. During her pregnancy, Jennifer attended one class related to the care of a newborn. "They taught us how to take a temperature and how we need to lay them down on their side when they are sleeping. My mom showed me how to give her a bath and take care of the umbilical cord."

SUBSTANCE USE

Your observation of the dirty ashtrays on the porch identifies the need for assessment related to substance (tobacco) use and second-hand smoke. This is a topic that was not identified as a priority in the previsit plan because there was no prior indication of smoking in the home.

When you mention the observation of ashtrays to the couple Joe states, "That's me, I know I shouldn't but I do smoke. We know it's not good for the baby so ever since we knew Jennifer was pregnant I've only smoked outside."

PROBLEM STATEMENT

Based on assessment data (subjective and objective information), how does your plan for nursing intervention differ from the previsit plan?

IDENTIFIED STRENGTHS

Your assessment has identified several sources of support for the family including both Jennifer and Joe's mothers. Before the visit you had no information about the couple's knowledge of nutrition, newborn care, or care of the perineal laceration. Your assessment has revealed the fact that the couple has received some information or training in the following areas:

- Perineal cleansing
- Postpartum vitamin supplementation
- Newborn care
  - Sleeping position
  - Bathing
  - Cord care
- Tobacco use and second-hand smoke
- Newly identified problems
  - Actual
    - Tobacco use
    - Knowledge deficit: nutrition
    - Knowledge deficit: care of newborn
  - Potential
    - Second-hand smoke

PLAN

At this point you must make necessary alterations in your preplan visit, considering your assessment data. Strengths have been identified. You now have important information about actual and potential problems and must develop your plan giving consideration to prioritizing the issues. Newly identified problems have been identified. By prioritizing the issues you can determine if your plan for this visit will include addressing newly identified problems.

NURSING INTERVENTION

PHYSICAL ASSESSMENT

During the physical assessment, it is important to:

- Make clients comfortable
- Teach clients how to assess and the significance of assessment
- How to identify variations, when to seek follow-up
- Wash hands before doing the assessment

Jennifer

- Vital signs
- Lochia
- Laceration
- Fundus

Clare

- Vital signs
- Nutritional status (weight)
- Reflexes
- Cord
- Jaundice (heel stick)
- Observe or ask about
  - Feeding patterns
  - Elimination
  - Sleeping patterns and position

Client education

Jennifer and Joe have related some knowledge about:

- Perineal cleansing
- Postpartum vitamin supplementation
- Newborn care
  - Sleeping position
  - Bathing
  - Cord care
- Tobacco use and second-hand smoke

Because the sources of information on the above topics are varied, it is wise to have Jennifer and Joe relate their knowledge of the subjects to you so that you may assess the accuracy of the information. This is also an opportunity to praise them for the acquisition of knowledge that will assist them in making the transition to parenthood.

At this time it is appropriate to review specific information related to prioritized topics:

1. Postpartum and newborn nutrition
2. Breast-feeding
3. Postpartum nutritional needs
4. Care of the newborn
5. Safety
6. Care of the perineal laceration

Appropriate referrals for this family may include:

- Transportation (ie, bus schedules, etc)

- Parenting classes
  - Family planning
  - Financial—AFDC
  - Low-cost child care resources
  - CPR/first aid courses
  - Nutritional—WIC

Planning for the second postpartum home visit should be a collaborative effort among Jennifer, Joe, and the nurse. Plans must be reasonable and must consider the limited time and resources of the clients.

Plan for second visit:

- Nurse
  - Bring information about
    Infant nutrition and developmental stages
  - Prepare for assessment of home
  - Explore other resources appropriate for needs of family
- Jennifer
  - Keep 3-day diet history
  - Write questions that come up between now and next visit
- Joe
  - Explore options for transportation

EVALUATION

The nurse determines if personal and group goals were met during this visit by discussing the visit with Joe and Jennifer. Together you will set mutual goals for subsequent visits. The goals of this visit, which were physical assessment of mother and newborn, basic psychosocial assessment of family with an emphasis on family dynamics, and health education, have been attained. Although in-depth assessment and teaching would have benefited this family, this will not be possible due to the limited number of visits. Ideally, appropriate and available community resources will assist in achieving this goal.

4.2 EXERCISE

DOMESTIC VIOLENCE ASSESSMENT

Please refer to 4.1 Case Study for case information.

Questions

1) Subjective and objective information: assessment. If Jennifer was physically abused by Joe, what types of cues (verbal and nonverbal)

might you have seen in the interaction with this family during your home visit?

2) Nursing intervention. How might your interaction have been different if you picked up on nonverbal cues by Jennifer that she wanted to have a private discussion with you and then revealed the fact that Joe had been physically abusive to her during the last trimester of her pregnancy?

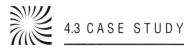 4.3 CASE STUDY

MEDICAL-SURGICAL: CEREBROVASCULAR ACCIDENT

SCENARIO

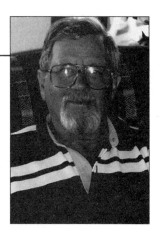

You are a discharge planner working for Capitol City Hospital. You will be providing patient education to a client, a 59-year-old man, who had a cerebrovascular accident (CVA) and will be discharged from the hospital and return home.

This client will be discharged at 3:00 PM; it is now 12:30 PM.

You have the following information regarding this client:

1) Sequelae of CVA include impaired mobility and impaired communication.
2) The client will be seen by his internist next week.
3) Prior to his CVA he was working as a chef in a large hotel.
4) His wife will be transporting him for his appointments.
5) Prescribed medications include anticoagulants and platelet aggregation inhibitors.
6) The client has a follow-up appointment in 3 days at Capitol City Hospital.

Questions

PLAN

1) Describe your plans for appropriate nursing interventions for this scenario.

2) State ways in which your plans may differ given the following situations:
   - The client will be discharged to Metropolis county jail; he was wanted on charges of fraud and placed under arrest shortly before his CVA.

   - The client is from the Philippines and speaks only Tagalog; you speak no Tagalog.

   - Nurses working with the client report to you that they have detected a strong odor of alcohol on his wife's breath during her visits with her husband.

   - The client is illiterate.

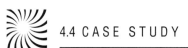 4.4 CASE STUDY

PRENATAL PLANNING AND INTERVENTION

SCENARIO

You are a public health nurse working the a prenatal clinic of Capitol City community

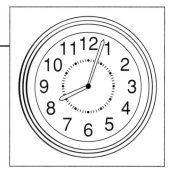

clinic. You are scheduled to see seven clients at this morning's prenatal clinic. Ms. Nolan is the first client. She has been examined by the physician, who has identified a discrepancy between the client's abdominal circumference and probable gestational age; the physician suspects intrauterine growth retardation. She asks you to order a sonogram for the client as soon as possible.

Ms. Nolan is entering her second trimester of pregnancy. This is her first prenatal examination. Her next prenatal visit will be in 4 weeks. If Ms. Nolan keeps all future scheduled visits, she will be seen approximately eight more times in your clinic. She sought prenatal care 3 weeks ago and was given an appointment for today. Some basic information was obtained from Ms. Nolan by telephone when she arranged for today's visit.

Ms. Nolan is a 25-year-old Anglo woman who is a single mother of three children, ages 10 months, 3 years, and 5 years. She is currently unemployed and receives Medicaid. She states that her maternal grandmother lives nearby and is very supportive. The grandmother assists with child care, transportation, diapers, and food.

On her intake questionnaire Ms. Nolan lists her primary concerns as:

- Exercise and weight control
- Housing options
- Birth control

Also notable from her interview is the fact that she reports having been sexually abused by her stepfather as a child. She stated that she has told very few people about this and has never sought counseling but feels she may be ready to discuss it at this point in her life.

Based on information from the interview with Ms. Nolan, along with clinic protocol, you have identified the following client needs:

1) Education about the glucose tolerance test that will be performed in 2 weeks
2) Education about laboratory testing to be performed, including human immunodeficiency virus (HIV) antibody and α-fetoprotein.
3) Discussion of client's desire for information about Lamaze classes
4) Further assessment of psychosocial situation
   a. Involvement of father of this child
   b. Family support other than grandmother
   c. Feelings about relationship with grandmother
5) Continued discussion of possible counseling resources
6) Discussion of desire for more children
   a. Family planning options—permanent, temporary
7) Prenatal nutrition
8) Prenatal exercise
9) Signs and symptoms warranting medical follow-up
   a. Fetal kick counts
10) Education about rationale and preparation for sonogram
11) Effects of the following on the fetus
    a. Alcohol

      b. Tobacco (ie, cigarettes, second-hand smoke)

      c. Drugs—illicit, prescription

12) Self-examination of breast

13) Infant growth and development

14) Labor and delivery

15) Preparing siblings

16) Preparing for breast-feeding

17) Safety measures specific to pregnancy

18) Community resources

      a. WIC

      b. Layettes

19) Self-care

      a. Prevention of urinary tract infections

      b. Kegel exercises

      c. Treatment of minor nausea, muscle soreness, fatigue

20) Birth plan

21) Review of laboratory and physical examination results

Questions

1) Identify other actual and potential problems.

2) Given the identified actual and potential problems, list them in order of priority and state rationale for this determination.

3) List actual and potential strengths.

4) You have 20 to 25 minutes to meet with Ms. Nolan in clinic today.
   - What additional assessment data will assist you in your interaction with Ms. Nolan?

  • What questions will you ask to elicit this information?

5) What issues will you address today?

  • Discuss your rationale for this approach.

6) What follow-up and referrals are appropriate and why?

7) How will you prioritize issues for subsequent visits?

8) What issues may not get addressed during the course of your relationship with Ms. Nolan? How does this make you feel?

4.5 EXERCISE

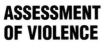

ASSESSMENT OF VIOLENCE

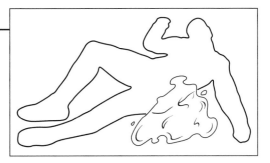

Violence is a major community health problem. State ways that a community health nurse, whose clients reside in a community with increasing levels of violence, might obtain valuable assessment data related to the following issues.

List potential resources for obtaining subjective and objective information (assessment data) related to each issue.

Issue	Resources for Subjective Data	Resources for Objective Data
Types of violent behaviors		
Incidence (numbers) of violent episodes		
Demographics of perpetrators		

Questions

1) Identify methods for reporting of violent activities.
   - Mandated reporting

   - Data collection methods

   - Agencies collecting data

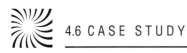

4.6 CASE STUDY

GERONTOLOGY

SCENARIO

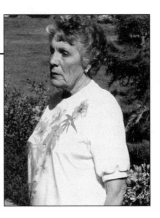

You are a nurse working for the home health agency in Brownsville. Your client is Mrs. Moberly, a 78-year-old Italian American woman. Mrs. Moberly had a myocardial infarction (MI) 2 weeks ago and was recently released from Brownsville Hospital. Home health nursing visits were prescribed by Mrs. Moberly's physician.

Three days ago you made your initial home visit with Mrs. Moberly. During this visit you discussed Mrs. Moberly's goals for home health nursing intervention. You asked her what she expected in terms of recovery rate and what her personal health goals are. You also assessed Mrs. Moberly's support system.

During your visit, you gathered some significant assessment data with which to plan subsequent visits with Mrs. Moberly.

Presented below are assessment data obtained from the client's medical record as well as from your initial visit. After reviewing the information presented below, state relevant issues and develop a plan of action for your involvement with Mrs. Moberly.

1. MD Rx
    a. Client to walk ½ to ¾ mile each day and to maintain heart rate not to exceed 105 beats per minute (bpm). Resting heart rate for Mrs. Moberly is 76 bpm
    b. Referral to be made to cardiac rehabilitation program at Brownsville Hospital
2. Rx also includes four to six visits by home health nurse for the following:
    a. Institution of exercise program—referral to occupational and physical therapy
    b. Management of therapeutic regimen—medications, diet, activity
3. Nursing assessment and instruction regarding personal monitoring of oxygen supply and demand, including activity tolerance
4. Assessment of home environment
    a. Safety
    b. Activities of daily living
5. Education about disease process
6. Sexual activity

Nursing Process

ASSESSMENT DATA

SUBJECTIVE

Mrs. Moberly lives alone in a small, older home in Brownsville. She has a daughter in town and a son living in Capitol City. Mrs. Moberly's daughter visits her every evening to assist her with bathing and laundry.

Before her MI, Mrs. Moberly enjoyed walking the two blocks to the community center for the senior citizen lunch program. Since her hospitalization she has not attended this program. She states that she has been fearful of venturing far from home due to her "condition" and adds that she finds herself easily fatigued when performing activities of daily living.

Mrs. Moberly states she has no questions or concerns about her medication regimen. She tells you that "since the tops are hard to open I just pour the pills on the counter. I can tell them apart by the way that they look." She adds, "I know the big round one I take in the morning when I wake up and then again before bed. The little blue one is supposed to be taken with meals."

Your client tells you that she has no questions about nutrition. "The doctor told me to cut back on salt and fat. I know all of that stuff. I raised two healthy children. I used to cook in my husband's restaurant . . . I know more than that young doctor about what's good for me."

OBJECTIVE

During your first visit with Mrs. Moberly you were greeted by an energetic, slightly built older woman. Although the home is small, there was sufficient room to walk about unobstructed. The furniture in the home appeared old but was in good condition. Two house cats were present during your visit.

You noticed soup cooking on the stove. Mrs. Moberly made no reference to the soup. It remained simmering on the stove for the length (55 minutes) of your visit.

Before this visit you drove the shortest route from the local community center to Mrs. Moberly's home. The distance to her home on the odometer read 0.2 of a mile.

Physical assessment during the initial visit revealed:

- Heart rate (resting): 85 bpm
- Respirations: 24
- Blood pressure: 138/77

Questions

STATEMENT OF CLIENT'S ISSUES
- Actual problems

- Potential problems

- Strengths
  - Actual

  - Potential

PLAN
- This visit
  - Additional assessment data to be gathered

- Subsequent visits

- Referrals

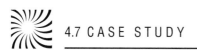 4.7 CASE STUDY

BACK PAIN

SCENARIO

You are hired as an occupational health nurse consultant by a cannery in Brownsville. The company's insurance rates have escalated because of an inordinate number of claims for back injuries. Injuries have included muscle spasms, lumbosacral strains, and intervertebral

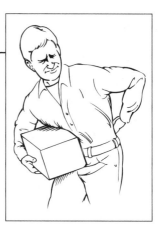

disk problems. You are contracted for 2 months of service. This is the first day of your assignment. Where do you begin?

Questions

1) What assessment data do you need?
   - Subjective

   - Objective

2) How will you go about gathering this information?

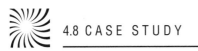 4.8 CASE STUDY

DRUG USE IN PREGNANCY

SCENARIO

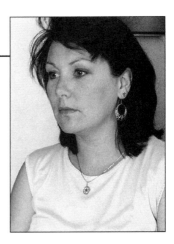

Your client is Zelda, a 32-year-old Anglo woman who is in her second trimester of pregnancy. She has received no prenatal care thus far in this pregnancy. Zelda lives in Smithville with the father of the baby, her boyfriend, who is also the father of her other children. She has three children, all of whom have been placed in foster care by the county social services agency. Zelda has a long history of injection drug use. She is currently participating in a methadone program in an attempt to "break" her heroin habit. Zelda has no family in the area. She is very involved in the local Narcotics Anonymous chapter and considers the members to be her "real family."

Zelda has informed you that her main objective at this time is "to get my 'act' together and get my kids back." Zelda receives food stamps and Social Security for a mental health disorder. She declines to discuss specific information about her mental health diagnosis.

Questions

Given this scenario, discuss your nursing interventions as you function in the following nursing roles:

1) You are a staff nurse on the medical-surgical unit of Brownsville Hospital. Zelda is one of nine patients for whom you have total nursing care responsibilities today. Zelda is being treated for an abscess on her right antecubital fossa; she is receiving intravenous antibiotics. Your supervisor has ranked her as having the lowest acuity among your patients. What is your focus for intervention with Zelda in this scenario?

2) You are a district public health nurse working in Smithville. A referral was made by children's protective services when they learned of the current pregnancy. You will be visiting Zelda, on a weekly basis, in her home. What is your focus for intervention with Zelda in this scenario?

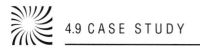 **4.9 CASE STUDY**

SEXUAL ASSAULT INVESTIGATION

SCENARIO

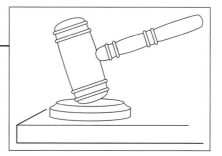

You are working as a sexual assault nurse examiner (SANE) in the emergency room (ER) of University Hospital in Metropolis. One evening a 17-year-old girl, Sheila, presents to the ER stating that she has been sexually abused by her stepfather. Two female friends have accompanied Sheila. Your role as a SANE requires you to be totally objective. Your job duties include data collection (subjective and objective) related to the alleged crime. You are also responsible for ensuring appropriate procedures are taken to maintain the integrity of all evidence. Additionally, in your role as a SANE you are not the advocate of the victim. You must be objective in your data collection to avoid bias.

The nursing process, as it applies to this scenario, through the implementation phase, will be presented here. You will be asked to discuss the evaluation phase of the nursing process given this scenario.

Assessment

SUBJECTIVE

Sheila states that this is the first incidence of sexual misconduct by her step-father. She reports that her mother is away on business this week and that she has been staying at home with her stepfather. She adds that the re-ported assault occurred at 7 that evening. Sheila reports having gone to bed at 9:30 and calling the two friends who have accompanied her to the ER. She states that they "convinced" her to allow them to drive her to the ER.

Specific information related to the alleged assault is related. The step-father reportedly approached Sheila while they were alone in the home. Sheila states that her stepfather was sitting next to her watching television. She adds that he "forced himself" on top of her and "pulled down my pants." She states that "he tried to go inside of me but I don't think he did; he was really drunk so when I screamed he got off of me and walked out of the house."

OBJECTIVE

Sheila presents at the ER at 11:50 PM. She is crying and holding on to the two friends who accompany her to the ER. Physical examination reveals the following:

1. No bruising or obvious trauma to the perineal area
2. Pubic hairs found and collected
3. Fibers found and collected
4. No semen found

Statement of the Issue

Seventeen-year-old female reporting sexual abuse by stepfather.

Plan

- Send for laboratory evaluation:
  - Hair
  - Fibers
  - Sexually transmitted diseases (including HIV), if warranted
- Photograph genital area for evidence of trauma.
- Ensure patient advocate is involved with the case as soon as possible.
- Ensure that all relevant subjective (victim's statements) and objec-tive (physical evidence) data are collected and sent to the appropri-ate authorities.
- Testify in pending court case.

Implementation

The client advocate was called within 4 minutes of Sheila's arrival to the ER. She arrived at the hospital 15 minutes later. Physical examination was begun after the client advocate arrived. Sheila was educated about the fol-lowing issues:

1. Role of the nurse as collector of information
2. Role of the advocate
3. Procedures necessary for data collection
4. Follow-up measures, both optional and recommended
   a. HIV antibody testing
   b. Testing for other sexually transmitted diseases (STDs)
   c. "Morning after" pill
5. Referrals made by advocate
   a. Psychological counseling
   b. Legal counseling
   c. Foster care

Data were collected per guidelines and included:

1. Documentation of Sheila's relevant statements
2. Physical evidence
   a. Microscopic
   b. Physical examination results—colposcopy

The trail of evidence was intact. Information was sent to appropriate agencies including mandatory reporting.

You testified at the trial regarding the results of the physical evidence. You received information about the results of the trial:

- The stepfather was found not guilty due to conflicting reports of his whereabouts at the time of the alleged sexual assault.

Questions

EVALUATION

1) Who was your client in this scenario?

2) What were the goals of your interaction with Sheila?

3) Did you do your job well?

4) Do you see yourself as an advocate in this scenario? To whom?

5) How might this scenario have differed if your job was ER staff nurse instead of SANE?
   - Were you uncomfortable with this scenario, with its subject matter?

   - What does your response to this scenario tell you about the role of SANE?

4.10 EXERCISE

ASSESSMENT TOOLS AND TECHNIQUES

Discuss ways in which the following tools and techniques may assist the community health nurse in gathering accurate and relevant assessment data regarding individuals and families in the environment of care.

Questions

1) Suggest scenarios in which these tools and techniques might be useful.

2) If you are unfamiliar with the tools listed below, discuss methods of obtaining additional information regarding their use and availability.

Tools and Techniques in Community Health Nursing

Tools
DDST (Denver Developmental Screening Test)
HOME (Home Observation for Measurement of Environment)
NCAST (Nursing Child Assessment Satellite Training)

(continued)

Tools and Techniques in Community Health Nursing (Continued)

Bayley Scale of Infant Development
Medical History/Admission Screening Test
Physical assessment • Height • Weight • Head circumference
Techniques
Reflective language
Empathy
Direct questioning
Open-ended questions
Identify tools available for community assessment

CHAPTER 5

Cultural Influences

"It is rare that one cannot learn from another or from life's experiences, if the effort is made. Perhaps that is the secret of achieving a peaceful society: searching for each other's unique and special knowledge."

Anonymous

"Knowledge is the antidote to fear."

Ralph Waldo Emerson

Chapter 5 presents information related to positive, negative, and neutral effects of culture on clients' health. The effects of culture on the practice of nursing are pervasive. In every area of practice, nurses must consider clients' culture when planning effective interventions. The field of community health nursing is particularly concerned with clients' culture because care is provided on clients' 'turf,' where cultural influences are more powerful than they might be in the hospital setting. Nurses' own culture has influence on, and is influenced by, the approach that they take with clients. Being aware of personal culture, as well as that of one's clients, will prepare nurses for effective practice in the community setting.

REVIEW

  I. Cultural assessment
     A. Self-assessment
         1. Cultural identity
         2. Ethnocentricity

    B. Assessment of cultural affiliations of client
       1. Appropriate questioning
       2. Active listening
    C. Tools of cultural assessment
       1. Individual
       2. Community
II. Gathering specific cultural information
    A. Examples of cultural groups and subgroups
       1. Religious groups
       2. Ethnic groups
       3. Homeless
       4. Poor
       5. Gangs
       6. Same-sex partners and families
       7. Immigrants
    B. Qualitative information related to cultural beliefs and values:
       1. Health
       2. Health care
       3. Illness causality
       4. Parenting
       5. Communication
       6. Family
       7. Age
       8. Education
       9. Use of community resources
      10. Nutrition
      11. Food
III. Significance of culture in community health nursing practice
    A. Developing and maintaining collaborative relationships
    B. Culturally sensitive patient teaching
    C. Effecting change within the cultural community
       1. Identifying leaders
IV. Transcultural nursing practice
    A. Theorist: Madeleine Leininger

DEFINITION

Culture: the lens through which individuals perceive and interact with themselves and the world around them

DISCUSSION

Much has been written about culture and its significance in nurses' interactions with clients. Nurses must be knowledgeable about cultural groups that they are likely to come in contact with in the performance of their job responsibilities. Nurses must be cognizant of the fact that as a member of a cultural group they possess beliefs and practices that may influence interactions with clients. Various types of cultural self-assessment tools are available to assist nurses in this process.

Although it is desirable that nurses increase their knowledge of diverse cultural groups, it is critical that this information is not generalized to all members of a cultural group. It is important to avoid making assumptions based on a client's cultural affiliation. Knowledge of clients' cultural affiliation is best used as a guide for effective application of the nursing process with individuals and aggregates.

Nurses use knowledge of a particular cultural group as a guide when interacting with members of that group. Such knowledge may be useful in identifying actual and potential client needs as well as strengths. The following considerations must be made when considering cultural influences of clients:

1. Culture is not synonymous with ethnicity.
2. Personal culture is often a 'blend' of various distinct cultural influences.
3. An individual may posses qualities of more than one cultural group.
4. There is great individual variation, even within clearly defined cultural groups.
5. Culture is a dynamic phenomenon.

Culture is a phenomenon learned from a group and reinforced by that group. Incorporating knowledge of a particular cultural group into the assessment phase of the nursing process, and listening to responses to nonjudgmental questioning, will provide the nurse with valuable data related to clients' cultural belief systems.

Cultural beliefs and practices may influence the health of the client in the following ways:

- Actual or potential negative impact
- No impact (innocuous or neutral)
- Positive impact

Case Studies and Exercises
APPROACH TO CASES AND EXERCISES

Cases and exercises have been written with no assumptions regarding the demographics of the learner. The questions should be approached by each student from the unique perspective brought by her or his own cultural identification.

Responses to the following case studies and exercises reflect the ability to:

1. Perform a cultural assessment.
2. Discuss the ways in which clients' culture influences their health status.

3. Based on a cultural assessment, identify information that is relevant for the nurse working in the community.
4. Discuss methods of gathering information regarding specific cultural groups.
5. Develop a culturally appropriate plan for nursing intervention.
6. Discuss ways in which personal culture may affect attitudes toward clients.
7. Identify gaps in knowledge regarding specific cultural groups.

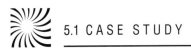 5.1 CASE STUDY

PEDIATRICS

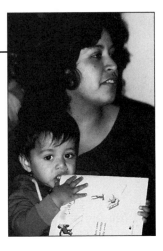

Given the following scenario, provide examples of questions that would elicit information about the client's cultural affiliations.

SCENARIO

You are a bilingual (Spanish and English) nurse practitioner working for a community clinic. In today's satellite clinic, you are performing well-child examinations for the population of a migrant farm labor camp in Smithville. Your client is Jasmine, the 20-month-old daughter of Mr. and Mrs. Espinoza. The family is monolingual, speaking only Spanish.

Mr. and Mrs. Espinoza express their concern about Jasmine's repeated ear infections. "We are always taking her into the emergency room in the middle of the night. She seems okay during the day and then she'll just wake up screaming." Mrs. Espinoza states that Jasmine has been seen in the emergency department twice in the past 4 months.

Your physical examination of Jasmine reveals normal growth and development with the exception of significant tooth decay ("bottle mouth"). Ears appear normal on examination today. You notice a bottle, with what appears to be chocolate milk, next to Jasmine in her stroller.

Questions

1) What do you need to know about this family?

2) How will you elicit necessary information?

The following information is necessary to identify possible etiologies of Jasmine's problems and to provide culturally sensitive education to her parents:

1) Detailed history of illnesses

2) Detailed history of treatments
> By family (home remedies)
> Prescribed by physician in emergency room
> History to include what was used, when, and with what results

3) Detailed dental history
> Onset of caries
> Previous treatment
> Prophylaxis
>> Fluoride
>> Brushing
>> Dental check-ups

4) Nutrition
> Child using bottle
> How often
> Contents of bottle
> "Propping"

5. Assessment of Jasmine's sleeping patterns prior to emergency room visits

Given the combination of "bottle mouth" and recurrent otitis media, you suspect the parents may be propping the child's bottle. Other factors may be contributing to Jasmine's identified problems. To gain information about factors relevant to Jasmine's health status you ask the following open-ended, culturally sensitive questions:

Questions	Client Responses
Who takes care of Jasmine most of the time?	Mrs. E: "I do, Mr. Espinoza works long hours in the field."
Who feeds Jasmine?	Mrs. E: "Mostly me, my oldest daughter helps out with the kids after school."
Who cooks the meals in your home?	Mr. E: "My wife, sometimes my mother brings something over. Also, the family eats alot of the fruits and vegetables that I bring from the fields."

(continued)

Questions	Client Responses
Describe a normal day's meals for Jasmine.	Mrs. E: "She eats the same as the rest of us . . . eggs, and potatoes in the morning, beans and tortillas at lunch and meat with tortillas and rice at night."
Does Jasmine enjoy her bottle?	Mr. E: "All of my kids loved their bottles."
What does Jasmine like to drink in her bottle?	Mrs. E: "Mostly juice and chocolate milk, sometimes aqua de aroz or manzanillo."
Why do you think she enjoys that type of drink?	Mrs. E: "I make sure she drinks the milk and juice, for her health."
When did you first notice that Jasmine was having problems with her ears?	Mr. E: "When she was about a year old."
What did you think was/is causing the problem?	Mr. E: "I think it's the cold air in our house, I keep telling the landlord to fix our heater, but it hasn't worked well since we moved there last year."
Have you tried any home treatment or remedy for Jasmine's ear problem?	Mrs. E: "Yes, I put the perfume in her ears and also an herb pack that my mother-in-law made for her."
Did the remedy work?	Mrs. E: "I think it made the fever go away and the ear didn't look so red, but she still woke up crying." "I think it didn't make the pain go away."
What medications has Jasmine been prescribed?	Mr. E: "They gave us some pink medicine when we took her to the doctor."
What have you been told about those medications?	Mr. E: "They said to give her the medicine until she felt better, so we did. Then she got sick again so we gave it to her again."
What do you think would help the problem with Jasmine's ears?	Mr. E: "This guy at my work said his boy had the same problems and the doctor put some tube in there and now he's all better, I think that might work."
How do Jasmine's teeth look to you?	Mrs. E: "All my kids' teeth looked like that, it's okay because it's just their baby teeth."

5.2 EXERCISE

PEDIATRICS ASSESSMENT

Refer to the scenario presented in Case Study 5.1 to respond to the following questions.

Using open-ended, nonjudgmental questions has provided you with important subjective and objective information about the influence of culture on this family.

Questions

1) List significant subjective and objective data that you have gathered from this interaction with the Espinoza family.
   * Subjective

   * Objective

2) How will you go about obtaining information about the following issues:
   * Hearing loss, speech development, and response to sounds
   * Balance and equilibrium
   * Exposure to second-hand smoke
   * Day care, exposure to other children
   * Diagnosis of chronic or periodic acute infection
   * Signs and symptoms of pain
   * Water exposure (bathing, swimming)

3) What constraints do time and potential for information overload have on your ability to perform a thorough assessment of this family?

4) How might your interaction with this family have been different if you were only English speaking and the parents were only Spanish speaking. Assume that your clinic has few monolingual Spanish-speaking clients and has no Spanish-English translators and that the family's 12-year-old nephew was brought along to translate.

5) Consider techniques you would use to integrate acknowledgment of this family's strengths in planning for nursing interventions.

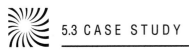 5.3 CASE STUDY

PEDIATRICS PLAN

Given the scenario presented in 5.1 Case Study, involving the Espinoza family, develop a plan for nursing intervention.

Questions

1) Given the information available to you, state identified cultural influences of the Espinoza family:
   - Negative influences

   - Potentially negative influences

- Neutral influences

- Positive influences

2) Prioritize the client and family needs.

3) Plan nursing interventions for this and subsequent visits to well-baby clinic (include patient teaching and referral plans).

5.4 E X E R C I S E

PSYCHIATRIC AND MENTAL HEALTH

Visualization

Scenario

You are grocery shopping late one evening in a busy area of town. You are alone. After making your purchases you enter the parking lot and walk toward your car. The parking lot is bustling with people getting in and out of their vehicles. You notice someone walking toward you from the center of the parking lot. You suspect it is a homeless person attempting to solicit a handout. You turn toward your car and see that the person turns in the same direction and attempts to make eye contact with you.

Reflections

Reader may ask questions and allow time for learners' quiet introspection.
1) How do you feel about this situation?

2) In your visualization how did this person look?
   - Age

   - Race

   - Gender

   - Hygiene

   - Clothing

3) What is the mental status of the individual in the parking lot?

4) Was the person under the influence of any substance? If so, what?

Questions

For group discussion
1) What presumptions did you make about the individual in the parking lot? What may have led to your preconceived notions?

2) Were your reactions "bad"? Why or why not?

3) What does this tell you about your cultural beliefs about the type of individual represented in this scenario?

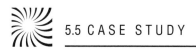 5.5 CASE STUDY

SEXUALLY TRANSMITTED DISEASE

SCENARIO

You are a nurse working in the sexually transmitted disease (STD) clinic in a community clinic in Capitol City. Your first client today is Lee, a 34-year-old Anglo man, who presents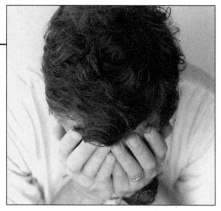
for follow-up evaluation of genital herpes. During his initial visit 2 weeks ago, he received education about its etiology and potential modes of infection.

Case Information

Lee presents today for a recheck. You review his understanding of medication administration and modes of transmission of the herpes virus. Lee relates accurate information about the disease process and reports compliance with prescribed medications. When asked about knowledge of modes of infection Lee becomes quiet and reserved, answering "yes or no" and avoiding eye contact. When you question him specifically about informing his wife of his infection he states "I have been meaning to but I just can't do it right now."

Having seen Lee during his initial visit to the STD clinic you are aware of the fact that he feels his infection was a result of a recent sexual relationship with a coworker. In the previous visit, he appeared anxious about his test results and made comments about how this would affect his image as a "good family man."

Questions

1) What is your initial reaction to Lee's situation?

2) Do you feel that your personal beliefs and values influenced your response to the scenario?

3) What reasons may the client have for his reaction?

4) What additional information will assist you in the provision of culturally appropriate education to this client?

5) What questions will you ask to obtain this information?

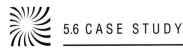 5.6 CASE STUDY

MEDICAL-SURGICAL

SCENARIO

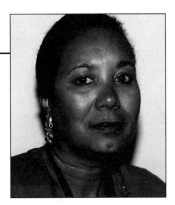

You are a nurse working for a nonprofit hospice agency. Your client is Justine, a 48-year-old Jamaican woman living in Brownsville. Justine was diagnosed with an inoperable brain tumor 3 months ago. She is receiving palliative treatment only and has been told she has a 4- to 6-month life expectancy. You have been her nurse for the past 2 months, making home visits two to three times each week. Sequelae of the illness and treatment include:

- Altered nutrition: less than body requirements related to fatigue
- Sensory-motor impairment
- Altered comfort: headaches

The purpose of your visits has been to assess Justine's physical and mental status, to assess efficacy of pain medication and level of pain, and to ensure adequate resources for nutrition, activities of daily living, and respite.

Justine is living with her partner of 6 years, Carla. Carla is an Anglo woman who works as a medical assistant for a local dermatologist. She is the primary caretaker for Justine but is gone 40 to 45 hours a week because of her job. She feels committed to maintaining this work schedule "because Justine is covered under my insurance policy as a domestic partner . . . I don't want to jeopardize my job because we can't afford to lose the insurance."

Justine has twin girls who attend college in Metropolis. Although the girls are aware of Justine's diagnosis, she has not discussed the details of the prognosis with them. "They have their own lives now, and I don't want to bother them with my problems," she states. Carla has no children. The couple had been politically active in the gay and lesbian community until the time of Justine's diagnosis. They have many friends who have maintained a supportive relationship with the couple.

Questions

1) List cultural influences that fall into the following categories:
   - Negative

   - Potentially negative

   - Neutral

   - Positive

2) What additional information may assist you in the provision and planning of care for this client?

3) What resources might assist the couple in the following areas:
   - Specific hospice services

- Psychosocial support (beyond hospice)

- Nutrition

- Home maintenance

4) What options might you discuss with Carla related to leave of absence from work?

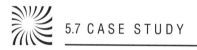 **5.7 CASE STUDY**

PAIN MANAGEMENT AND CAREGIVER STRESS

Please refer to 5.6 Case Study.

PAIN MANAGEMENT

Discuss your feelings regarding pain management in clients with terminal illness.

Justine and Carla have identified pain management as their primary concern. As a hospice nurse, what pharmacologic, physical, and cognitive approaches to pain management might you use in your interactions with this couple?

CAREGIVER STRESS

Discuss potential stressors affecting Carla as the primary caretaker for Justine.

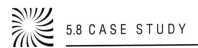 5.8 CASE STUDY

REPETITIVE USE INJURY

SCENARIO

You are an occupational health nurse working for a computer firm in Metropolis. Your client is Mr. Singh, who was referred to you for evaluation and follow-up of possible carpal tunnel syndrome. Mr. Singh is a data entry clerk for the company. Your job is to evaluate work conditions that may be contributing to the problem and to refer Mr. Singh to a specialist for evaluation and follow-up of the existing condition. You will also be involved in any necessary retraining recommendations for Mr. Singh.

Your company works exclusively with a physical therapy group run by an orthopedist, Dr. Raj. Your plan is to have Dr. Raj evaluate Mr. Singh and identify diagnosis and recommended follow-up therapy. You will work with Mr. Singh to schedule appointments that will not conflict with his work schedule.

Mr. Singh comes to your office immediately after his initial visit with Dr. Raj and states "I will not work with that man . . . he is a Hindu and I don't feel comfortable with him." After questioning Mr. Singh further you discover that he is of the Sikh religion, which has animosity toward members of the Hindu religion. Mr. Singh feels that although Dr. Raj seemed pleasant enough, he does not want him as his physician.

Questions

1) What is your initial reaction to this situation?

2) What additional information might assist in the development and possible revision of your plan of care for this client? How will you obtain this information?

3) Will you involve the physician (Dr. Raj) in the planning process?

4) What is your responsibility as the occupational health nurse for the company?

5) Does Mr. Singh have a right to special treatment, including the expense of a noncontracted physician? Why or why not?

6) What are your options in this situation?

5.9 EXERCISE

HEALTH BELIEFS AND PRACTICES

Questions

1) List five distinct cultural groups living in your community.

2) Present practices or belief systems held by the group that may influence their health and well-being.

Group	Positive Effect on Health	Negative Effect on Health
1		
2		
3		
4		
5		

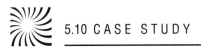 5.10 CASE STUDY

ADULT DAY HEALTH PROGRAM

SCENARIO

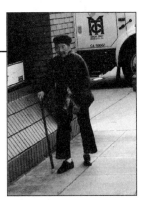

You have accepted a position as the supervising nurse in an adult day health program in Metropolis. The previous supervisor left the position under duress, amidst complaints by clients and their family members. It was felt that the previous supervisor was culturally insensitive, that the education and services provided at the center did not meet the needs of the population. Health department administrators were told by clients and family members that the supervisor "made them feel bad," that "they thought they were bad because they couldn't do all of the things that she told them about changing their diet and exercising . . . it was like they were being blamed for being old and sick."

Clients reportedly felt that "some of the things they asked us to do were uncomfortable and embarrassing." Most notable was the fact that offense was taken at the manner in which the previous program director dealt with the issues of breast self-examinations for men and women and prostate examinations for men. Clients reported feeling embarrassed discussing these issues in a group setting.

Health Program Data

The adult day health program and its clients have the following characteristics.

Population

Number of clients served: 68

Age range: 65 to 102

Ethnicity: 60% African American, 30% Anglo, and 10% Asian

Income level: income at or below poverty level qualifies individuals for this free program; many clients have Medicare

Medical issues: varied, numerous chronic health problems such as:

- Hypertension
- Diabetes mellitus
- Emphysema
- Chronic obstructive pulmonary disease/congestive heart failure
- Inflammatory joint disease
- Obesity
- Cataracts
- Macular degeneration
- Cancer
- Postcerebrovascular accident

Staffing: You supervise one licensed vocational nurse and two medical assistants.

Administered by: County Health Department

Funding: Older Americans Act, City of Metropolis

Program goals:

- Nutrition services
- Health assessment
  - Blood pressure screening
  - Foot checks
  - Weight
  - Eyesight
- Health education
  - Exercise
  - Nutrition
  - Safety
- Resource education
  - Insurance programs
  - In-home services
  - Financial assistance and planning
- Guest speakers
- Social programs
  - Cards, games, entertainment

Questions

1) Cultural self-awareness
   - How would you characterize the culture of the group attending the program?

   - Do you feel that you possess sufficient knowledge of these cultural groups to perform effectively if you were to 'step in' to the role of program supervisor?

2) Given this group's experience with the previous program director, it is imperative that you ensure that cultural relevance and sensitivity are incorporated into the program.
   - State methods that you will use to assess the following issues related to the group's cultural belief system.
   - Be specific about the language and type of questions to be used.
   - List individuals and groups that may assist you by providing relevant assessment data.
   - How will you assess the following (Gagnon, 1983, p. 130):

Issues	*Assessment*
Value systems • Beliefs • Taboos	
Goals and expectations	
Definition of health	
Values and attitudes toward health	
Existing preventive health behavior	

(continued)

Issues	Assessment
Perception of health problems	
Acceptability of health programs	
Perception of the purpose of health programs	

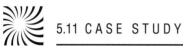

5.11 CASE STUDY

MEDICAL-SURGICAL

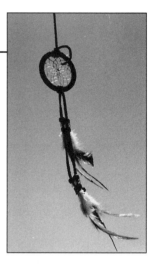

SCENARIO

As a hospice nurse in Brownsville, you have worked with diverse cultural groups. Presented below is a case that has challenged you to reflect on your cultural awareness.

Your client is Betsy, a 32-year-old woman with end-stage ovarian cancer. Betsy is divorced and lives on a ranch on the outskirts of Brownsville. She has two daughters, ages 9 and 11. She and her children moved to Brownsville from Alaska 5 years ago, following the divorce. Her extended family lives in Alaska.

After initial attempts at treatment using alternative medical therapies, Betsy sought the services of an oncologist. Surgery was performed and the tumor was removed, but the cancer had metastasized. Betsy underwent intensive chemotherapy and radiation therapies after surgery. Despite her efforts, the use of both conventional and alternative medical practices, interventions aimed at curing the cancer were unsuccessful. She has been told by her physician that she has less than 6 months to live.

Betsy had many long discussions with both her oncologist and her shaman. Although her oncologist offered to continue treatment using more aggressive therapies, Betsy decided to discontinue all methods of conventional treatment. She has requested the use of medication, at her discretion, as a palliative measure. She informed her physician that her shaman had assisted her in her decision and that she wanted to spend as much quality time as possible with her children. She stated that she felt that her decision to forgo aggressive therapies would allow her to achieve this goal.

When Betsy decided to discontinue all therapies except palliative, your hospice agency became involved in her care and you were assigned as Betsy's nurse. You have made three visits to the family's home and feel that you have begun to develop a trusting relationship with Betsy and have become close to her and her daughters.

To effectively work with Betsy and her girls through the process of death and dying, it is imperative that you become familiar with their cultural beliefs and practices. Based on reports from previous health care providers, along with assessment data gathered through your observations and discussions in the family's home, you are aware of the fact that Betsy practices alternative medicine. She has made references to her shaman as well as an herbalist who has assisted her with remedies for insomnia. Additionally, Betsy has voiced her frustration regarding traditional medical practices. "I wish I had never gone to that doctor," she stated. "I feel like maybe if I'd stuck with what I really believe in I wouldn't be in this situation."

Because you do not have specific information about the family's cultural beliefs related to health, illness, and dying, you determine that a cultural assessment is warranted at this time.

The goals of the assessments include:

1. Increase your knowledge of the family's:
   - Beliefs about death
   - Beliefs about pain
   - Plan for death and dying
   - Goals for your (hospice) intervention
   - Spiritual beliefs about death and dying
     - Assess for spiritual needs during and after death
2. Identify potential resources (in addition to hospice) that may assist the family.
3. Determine hospice resources to be used.
4. Determine alternative medicine resources available locally.
5. Determine the extent to which traditional medical practices are accepted and desired (ie, pain medications).
6. Identify plans for the girls:
   - During the dying process
   - At the time of death
   - After Betsy's death
7. Assure the family that they can openly discuss their beliefs and desires with you.
   - Clarify your role along with the services you may offer.

Questions

1) Perform a cultural assessment of Betsy and her family using the role-play format.

Role Play: Cultural Assessment

Nurse	*Betsy*

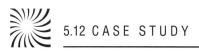 5.12 C A S E   S T U D Y

COMMUNICABLE DISEASE

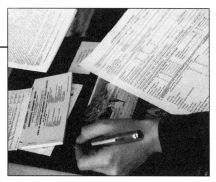

SCENARIO

You are a nurse working for the Brownsville Department of Health. One of your responsibilities is epidemiologic follow-up on reports of communicable disease. Today you will be performing your second visit on the following clients:

Tai: a 17-year-old boy

Nguyen: a 15-year-old girl

Tai and Nguyen are cousins. Both clients became infected with *Salmonella* from undercooked pork after a church picnic. Both are from Vietnamese families who immigrated to the United States 7 years ago.

During your initial visit, you spoke with the parents of Tai and Nguyen and educated them about the following:

1. Medication administration
2. Strict handwashing
3. Proper bowel habits
4. Food preparation and handling
5. Treatment of gastrointestinal sequelae
6. Collection of stool specimens
7. Modes of transmission
8. Assessment indicating exacerbation of signs and symptoms

The information you presented related to *Salmonella* was taken from recommendations from the Board of Health. In your education of the parents, you were careful to impress on them the potential deleterious consequences of noncompliance with these standards. You warned them that other family members would be placed at risk if there was deviation from the recommended practices.

On your return visit today, you are presented with the following scenarios:

1. Tai's family has followed your directions meticulously. His father tells you that the family has declined an invitation to an upcoming church social "because they're the ones who made my boy sick . . . they don't cook things right and I'm not taking my family there anymore," he states. The parents also advise you that they have stopped giving Tai herbal teas and are instead providing him with rehydration drinks as recommended by his physician.

   Additionally, Tai's parents have prohibited their children from visiting their cousins "because they don't take good care of themselves." Tai's mother tells you, "their kids don't even wash their hands after using the toilet and you said that would make us all sick."

2. Your visit with Nguyen and her parents reveals the following information. Nguyen has refused to provide a stool specimen. Her parents speak little English and rely on Nguyen for interpretation. "They think you were mad at them last time," Nguyen informs you. "They got upset and scared." Nguyen goes on to tell you that "we're not drinking that stuff you told us about. . . . My mom says that the tea has worked for our people for generations so it's good enough for me." Nguyen adds that her parents have used spooning techniques to provide her with relief from gastrointestinal problems.

Questions

1) Is there a 'good' and a 'bad' client in this scenario?

2) Did you achieve desired nursing outcomes based on your intervention with Tai's family? Why or why not?

3) What might you have done differently to ensure the provision of culturally appropriate education with these families?

4) How might mutual goals have been developed?

Reference

Gagnon, A.T. (1983). Trans cultural nursing: Including it in the curriculum. *Nursing and Health Care, 4*(2), 127–131.

CHAPTER 6

Systems Theories

Nurses in the community work with and within many types of systems. Effective and efficient community health nursing practice requires an understanding of, and an ability to work with and within, these systems. The systems to which community health nurses will relate may vary from those encountered by nurses working in the acute care system. Chapter 6 reviews the effects of clients' systems on their health practices and health status. Various types of systems, their components, and their boundaries are discussed.

REVIEW

- I. Definitions
   - A. General
   - B. Nursing
   - C. Holism
- II. Types of systems
   - A. Open or closed
   - B. Personal, interpersonal, and societal
   - C. Dynamic or static
- III. Theorists
   - A. Imogene King
   - B. Dorothy Johnson
   - C. Betty Neuman
   - D. Sister Callista Roy
- IV. Systems in community health
   - A. Individual
   - B. Family
   - C. Agency

    D. Community
    E. Professional
 V. Theories: family systems
    A. Theoretical concept: family dynamics
      1. Family developmental theory
      2. Family developmental framework
    B. Functions of the family (Spradley, 1996, p. 355)
      1. Affection
      2. Security and acceptance
      3. Identity and satisfaction
      4. Affiliation and companionship
      5. Socialization
      6. Controls
    C. Developmental tasks of families
    D. Social structure of families
      1. Family unit
      2. Individual members
        a) Power structure
          (1) Decision makers
        b) Boundaries
        c) Types of family structure
          (1) Traditional
          (2) Nuclear
          (3) Nuclear dyad
          (4) Single parent
          (5) Single adult
          (6) Multigenerational
          (7) Dual career
        d) Nontraditional
          (1) Commune
          (2) Group marriage
          (3) Unmarried couple
          (4) Same-sex partners
          (5) Nonrelated adults ("friends")
          (6) Nonsexual relationship
        e) Biologic versus chosen families
    E. Communication of the family
      1. Patterns
        a) Triangulation
      2. Styles
    F. Family belief system
      1. Health
    G. Culture
    H. Family health assessment
      1. Data collection techniques
        a) Tools

  2. Risk factors of family
      a) Group
      b) Individual
  3. Strengths
  4. Problems
  5. Resources
  6. Personal
  7. Community
I. Vulnerable family systems
  1. Dysfunctional family systems

DISCUSSION

Family Systems

- Why is it important for the community health nurse to have an understanding of the dynamics of the client's family?

An understanding of family dynamics enhances the community health nurse's opportunity for successful interaction with families. Identifying power structures within families, cultural influences, beliefs about health and illness, and other relevant issues are all important aspects of data collection related to family dynamics.

Understanding the role of the identified client within the family system is accomplished through the use of family assessment tools and techniques. Such information will assist the nurse in developing a plan for holistic care of the individual, given the unique characteristics of the particular family system. In identifying and working toward mutual goals, the community health nurse who is aware of the family's perception of the individual client, and his or her related health and illness issues, may work within the boundaries of the family's belief system to effect change. Similarly, in situations in which the belief system of the family has deleterious effects on the health and well-being of the client, the nurse who has performed an assessment of the family dynamics is equipped to work with the client and family toward identification and achievement of mutually identified goals.

- How does the community health nurse elicit information about family dynamics?

Several excellent data collection tools (see pp. 84–85) are available for use in the community setting. Agencies providing health care services in the community setting have an obligation to educate staff about tools that are available and relevant for the populations they serve. Ensuring competency in use of these tools is the joint responsibility of the employing agency and the community health nurse. Nurses must continue to use general nursing assessment techniques such as goal-directed questioning and active listening. These skills provide the basis for effective data collection.

Empathic, nonjudgmental responses by the nurse will encourage families to be forthright in their discussions. Such responses are more likely to provide the health care team with accurate subjective assessment data. The community health nurse must have the skills and knowledge base that creates an environment conducive to self-disclosure on the part of the client and family system.

Objective data related to the family system are obtained by observation of family interactions as well as the client's milieu. Nurses must be educated about nonverbal communication, such as body language, to make accurate assessments based on objective data. By applying appropriate theoretical concepts, the nurse makes determinations about family function based on subjective and objective assessment data.

- What techniques might the community health nurse use to involve the family in the care of the client?

Focusing on the positive aspects of the family system is an effective means of enlisting families in the nurse–client interaction. Identifying and using families' strengths allows the nurse to observe and assess optimal functioning of the family system. Additionally, identification of the family's internal resources demonstrates confidence in the family's ability to influence the situation. Encouraging families to access available and appropriate external resources promotes the independence of the family system from temporary support systems such as the community health nurse.

Allowing for decision making on the part of the individual client, in conjunction with his or her family, assists in the development of realistic mutual goals. The appropriate degree of involvement of the client's family members depends on several factors, including the medical and psychological status of the client, the client's desire for family involvement, and the family's desire and ability to participate in the care and maintenance of the client's needs. The nurse must make every effort to ensure that the client is an active participant in the planning and implementation of care. A holistic approach involving family members, to the degree deemed appropriate by the client and nurse, will likely result in improved client outcomes.

- Traditional versus nontraditional families

The terms traditional and nontraditional family are used to classify various types of living situations found in society. Nursing assessment of the family structure may lead to the conclusion that the client's family structure has well-defined boundaries that meet the specific criteria for one category of family structure. Frequently, however, clients' living situations are a combination of one or more categories or in a state of flux.

It is important to understand that the term "traditional" is not synonymous with "normal." Living situations previously considered "nontraditional" are becoming more common. This may be due in part to a shift in cultural norms and mores. In addition, families who previously may have been reluctant to discuss personal living situations with others, including the community health nurse, may experience less stigma attached to their situation and therefore be more open about discussing such issues.

Agency, Community, and Professional Systems

Nurses' relationships with systems in the community are equally important as those with the client system. To be effective in implementing change within family systems, the nurse must have a good understanding of, and be skilled at interacting with, external systems influencing the health of clients and their families. Nurses' roles have changed dramatically as a result of health care reform. This period of change presents nursing with the challenge and the opportunity to define its role in collaborative practice.

A major goal of health care reform is the provision of health care that is efficient, nonfragmented, and patient focused (Wolf, Boland, & Aukerman, 1994, p. 54). To achieve this goal, health care practitioners must develop, and strive to maintain, professional working relationships. Responsibilities of health care providers must be clearly delineated to avoid overlap and confusion. Wolf and colleagues (1994, p. 55) describe four concepts supporting collaborative practice:

- Professional communications: verbal and nonverbal interactions that define the relationships
- Unit norms: accepted formal and informal rules that govern interactions that may or may not be consistent with the organization's culture
- Professional shared governance: a structure to support collaboration among professionals in determining standards for the professional practice of nursing
- Interdisciplinary relationships: the interaction of the roles of the various members of the healthcare teams.

Skills that will assist the community health nurse in developing successful working relationships with agencies, communities, and colleagues are similar to those necessary to work effectively with family systems. These skills include:

1. Identifying the system's:
   Components
   Boundaries
   External influences
   "Key players" or "power brokers"
   Weaknesses or gaps
2. Focusing on the strengths and abilities of the system
3. Determining functional ability prior to delegation of follow-up activities

Case Studies and Exercises

Responses to the following case studies and exercises reflect the ability to:

1. Perform an assessment of a particular system.

2. Based on the assessment of the system, identify the system's boundaries, members, dynamics, and external and internal influences.
3. Discuss skills that, when used effectively by the nurse, can promote a higher level of functioning by a system.
4. Give examples of factors that influence individuals as open systems.
5. Explain which interventions would be most effective given the dynamics of a particular system.
6. Discuss the impact of a system's activities on the health of its members.

6.1 EXERCISE

SELF-ANALYSIS

Using the lines intersecting the circle, list factors that exert influence over you as an individual and an open system (ie, specific individuals, organizations, work).

1. Place your name inside the circle.
2. Think about the type and degree of influence that each of these factors has on you as an open system.
3. Be prepared to discuss your responses with a peer.

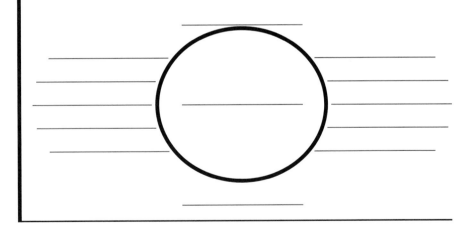

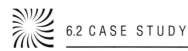 6.2 CASE STUDY

HOMELESSNESS AND TUBERCULOSIS

SCENARIO

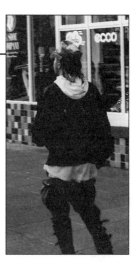

You are a nurse working for the juvenile detention center in Metropolis. Your client is Steven, aged 17, who is incarcerated for armed robbery. Steven has served 16 months of an 18-month sentence. Recently, Steven received a tuberculin skin test that demonstrated a positive reaction. During the period of Steven's incarceration, there was a case of active TB in juvenile hall. You are following up with Steven today for a positive tuberculin skin test and a negative chest x-ray. Additionally, the jail physician has prescribed isoniazid daily for 6 months as a prophylactic measure.

Steven was living on the streets before his incarceration. He left home at the age of 15. Steven's father is a severe alcoholic who was physically and emotionally abusive to Steven. Steven's mother was also physically abused by this man. Before leaving home, Steven attempted to convince his mother to leave but she refused. Steven has no siblings and is estranged from his extended family. He states that his 'family' now is his gang, a group of teens living on the streets who support themselves by panhandling and petty theft.

Steven tells you about his life on the streets. He informs you that his 'family' travels around quite a bit and that they live in a renovated school bus. He adds that although they have "been hassled" by the police, they are not involved in violent activities. He does admit that the group "likes to smoke weed a lot . . . but that just makes us mellow."

Your goal for Steven is that he have an understanding of the importance of TB prophylaxis and that he continue taking his medication after his release from juvenile hall. You would like to ensure that he have an understanding of the signs and symptoms of TB and appropriate follow-up measures should a problem arise.

Questions

1) List family system issues that you must consider when planning for Steven's release from juvenile hall.

2) Using systems theories, brainstorm about appropriate methods of education for Steven.

3) List specific ways in which you may work to increase Steven's chances of adhering to the prescribed medication regimen after his release from the detention center.

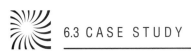 6.3 CASE STUDY

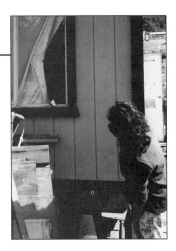

MEDICAL-SURGICAL: SPINAL CORD INJURY

SCENARIO

You are a home health nurse working in Smithville. You have been given a referral for a new client, Hector. Hector is being released from the rehabilitation unit of Metropolis Hospital. Although he lives in Smithville, Metropolis Hospital was the only facility willing to accept a Medicaid client with a severe spinal cord injury.

Hector is a 19-year-old Hispanic man who sustained major injury to his spinal cord (T-4 injury) in a motorcycle accident. The injury occurred approximately 6 weeks ago. Hector has been diagnosed as paraplegic with some residual limitation of upper body strength and mobility.

Your job is to facilitate Hector's transition from the hospital to the home environment. You will be teaching Hector and his caregivers about the following:

1. Nutrition and fluid intake
2. Signs and symptoms warranting follow-up
3. Medication administration
4. Bowel and bladder care
5. Skin care
6. Activities of daily living (ADLs), self-care with sensory-motor deficits
7. Safety and injury prevention
8. Community resources
9. Rehabilitative services

10. Anticipatory guidance regarding
    - Grief, anger, and suicidal ideations
    - Sexual function
    - Fear of abandonment, role change, and social isolation
    - Altered family processes

Following is a synopsis of information obtained during your initial visit with Hector and his family in their home.

Visit One

Hector lives in a migrant labor camp located on the outskirts of Smithville. His family has resided in the camp for 18 years. Living in the two bedroom cabin-like home are:

- Hector
- Hector's uncle, Manuel (32 years old)
- Hector's brother, Efran (16 years old)
- Manuel's wife, Micaela (29 years old)
- Manuel and Micaela's children, Arturo (5 years old) and Jasmin (6 months old)
- Hector's 74-year-old paternal grandmother (Abuela) who has recently arrived from Mexico and plans on assisting in Hector's care

The whereabouts of Hector's mother are unknown; she moved from their village in Mexico shortly after Efran was born. She has remarried and started another family. She has had no contact with Hector or Efran. Hector's father lives in their home village in Mexico. Although he lived in the migrant camp in Smithville for many years, he recently remarried and has two young daughters in Mexico. Hector's father is aware of Hector's injury and has no plans to return to the United States.

Your ability to speak fluent Spanish has enabled you to elicit the above information. Manuel has provided you with most of the information. He has been very involved in Hector's recovery, through daily visits to the rehabilitation unit and frequent discussions with Hector's health care providers. Manuel tells you that "Hector is like a son to me . . . I have a responsibility to my older brother to watch over his son. My brother watched out for me when I was young . . . he even left school to work to help support our family." Manuel adds, "We don't have much but we will take care of Hector . . . we'll all work together."

You begin your discussion by explaining your role as home health nurse. You inform the family about the type of education and interventions you are able to provide. You ask Hector and the family to tell you what they have learned from the health care team at the rehabilitation unit and what plans have been developed by the family to address Hector's medical and psychosocial needs. As you begin the visit, you notice that Hector's grandmother is sitting quietly in a corner of the room rocking Jasmin. You learn that Efran is working in the fields. Arturo is in school. Manuel, Micaela, and Abuela are participating in the home visit this morning.

The conversation is as follows:

Nurse	*Client/Family*
Hector, can you tell me how you feel about being home?	(*Hector* looks at Micaela) Okay I guess. (*Micaela*) He's a little scared I think, he feels like its going to be too much for us to deal with.
(looking at Hector) There's so much happening right now, so much to think about . . .	(*Hector*) Uh-huh.
(Hector is maintaining eye contact with Manuel and Micaela only; since this is your initial visit to the home you feel that Hector may be more comfortable in the role of observer).	
(looking at Manuel and Micaela) Do you have any questions before we begin?	(*Micaela*) They gave us alot of information at the hospital . . . I'm most afraid about if the phone doesn't work and Hector needs help . . . what if something happens to Hector and I can't call anyone . . . that's the only thing I worry about. (*Abuela*) If anything happens to him I'll be right here with you 'mija'. We can do this, we can take care of Hector if we work together. (*Manuel*) There is a store with a phone only two blocks away, if you needed to you could call from there. What I want to know is how we can get Hector into school or something that will help him be around kids his own age. His English is good enough, he even finished high school. He needs to be ready to make a future for himself. (*Hector* grins and looks at Manuel) Right uncle, that is what I want too.

You continue the conversation by revisiting Micaela's concerns about access to a telephone in case of an emergency. You ask specific questions about her concerns and use this as an opportunity to educate the family about circumstances warranting immediate follow-up. Together you decide that Micaela will develop a list of specific concerns that you will review together at a subsequent visit planned for 2 days from today.

Today's visit consists of:

1. Assessment
   - Home environment
     - safety
     - ADLs
   - Knowledge of disease processes
   - Fluid volume balance
   - Nutritional resources of family
     - Food availability
     - Food preparation
   - Insurance and financial status
2. Education
   - Medications
   - Warning signs and symptoms and appropriate follow-up procedures
   - Bowel and bladder care
   - Hygiene before and after patient care

The plan for your visit in 2 days includes:

1. Referrals
   - Community resources
   - Educational opportunities
   - Support groups (Spanish speaking)
   - Peer group opportunities for Hector
2. Assessment
   - Continuation of above
3. Education
   - Continuation of above

Questions

1) What is the social structure of this family (traditional versus nontraditional)? Be specific about the type of traditional or nontraditional family system that exists in this scenario.

2) Discuss an example of triangulation in this scenario.

3) What essential functions are present within this family system?

4) What developmental stages appear to have been achieved?

5) What steps will you take to empower the family to make its own decisions?

6.4 EXERCISE

HEALTH CARE SYSTEMS

You are a supervising nurse in a nonprofit community clinic located in Brownsville. The clinic provides health care services to a large Korean immigrant population in central Capitol City. Many of the clients receiving services from the clinic are undocumented immigrants. A recent crop failure has eliminated many of the warehouse jobs held by clients and their families. For the undocumented aggregate, no unemployment or Medicaid benefits are available to hold them over until other employment opportunities arise.

These problems have led to increasing numbers of clients presenting with little or no financial resources to pay for the health care services provided at the clinic.

The members of a health care team working in the clinic are listed inside of the circle representing an open system. Using the lines entering the open system, list factors in this scenario that have, and may, influence the agency and the health care team.

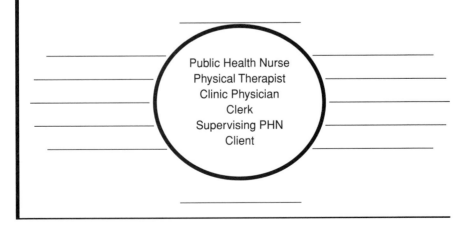

Public Health Nurse
Physical Therapist
Clinic Physician
Clerk
Supervising PHN
Client

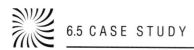 **6.5 CASE STUDY**

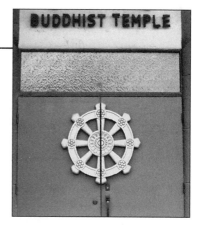

GERONTOLOGY

SCENARIO

You work as a liaison between a group of privately owned skilled nursing facilities (SNFs) and a large home health agency in Metropolis. Your job involves coordination of discharge planning for clients from SNFs to their homes and determination of optimal (home versus SNF) placement for clients. This determination is based on client preference, home environment, family support, and financial (cost–benefit) analysis.

Your client is the Hu family. Mr. Hu is a 79-year-old man who has been in the SNF of Metropolis Hospital for the past 2 months, following surgery for bilateral total hip replacement (arthroplasty). Although his recovery has been slower than anticipated, SNF staff and Mr. Hu's physician feel that he is now ready for transition to the home environment. He will need these follow-up services:

1. Home health nursing services for
   - Wound care
   - Assessment of home safety and self-care
   - Education about
     - Medications
     - Nutrition (including weight control)
     - Prevention of colonic constipation
     - Signs and symptoms of complications: fat emboli, hemorrhage, infection, dislocation
     - Mobility/ambulation with assistive device for altered gait
2. Occupational health nursing services in the home
3. Physical therapy services in the home
4. Caregiver assessment and training
5. Rehabilitative program
6. Community resources

Both Mr. and Mrs. Hu speak only Cantonese. They have had little contact with individuals outside their cultural circle in the Buddhist community. On the rare occasions when they have needed assistance with English, they have relied on their granddaughter, their son, or members of their temple. The type of home interventions that will be performed by the home health nurse, occupational health nurse, and physical therapist will all require a great deal of verbal communication with the Hus.

Mr. and Mrs. Hu reside in a middle-class neighborhood in suburban Metropolis. They have a close network of friends and family and are very involved in the Buddhist community in the city. They have one child, a son named Kwon. Their son lives in Metropolis and works as a computer programmer. He works long hours, often in excess of 10 hours per day. Although he is emotionally supportive and frequently calls his parents from work during the day, he is not available for assistance on weekdays due to the demands of his job. Kwon has a 15-year-old daughter named Leanne who lives with her mother in Metropolis. Although Kwon is divorced, Leanne maintains a close relationship with her paternal grandparents. Leanne spends two to three afternoons per week at the home of Mr. and Mrs. Hu. She is unsure if this tradition will continue given her grandfather's return home and his need for recuperation.

Questions

In anticipating the needs of the Hus, consider the following issues related to support systems of this family.

1) What support might be available through the agencies working with the Hus?

2) What type of support is available within the family system?

3) What external supports seem appropriate for assistance in this scenario?

4) How might you maximize the resources available to arrange for appropriate follow-up care and education for the Hus?

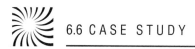 6.6 CASE STUDY

USE OF TRANSLATOR

Please refer to 6.5 Case Study.

SCENARIO

You have scheduled a visit with Mr. and Mrs. Hu. No family member is available to translate and therefore you have scheduled a bilingual (English–Cantonese) community health worker from your agency to meet you at the home to provide translation services.

In previous visits you addressed many of the needs facing this family and feel that you have established trust and developed rapport. Among the items you planned on assessing today are concerns or questions regarding sexual functioning.

You begin by reviewing the physician's recommendation regarding activity. You advise the couple that according to Mr. Hu's physician, sexual activity will have no adverse affect on Mr. Hu's current medical condition. You encourage the couple to feel free to ask you any questions they may have regarding the subject of sexual activity. After you have presented the data to the translator and asked her to relay the information, you watch the couple for their response. You are surprised when the translator's dialogue is brief and Mr. Hu responds with a single word response. The translator advises you: "They don't have any questions about that, they say everything is okay with that stuff."

Questions

1) What, if any, actual or potential problems do you identify in this interchange?

2) What actions might you have taken before the visit to ensure appropriate translation services?

3) What actions might you take at this juncture to ameliorate the situation?

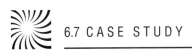 **6.7 CASE STUDY**

DIABETES

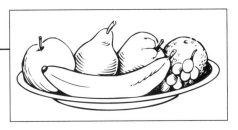

SCENARIO

As the supervising nurse on the
evening shift in Capitol City jail, you review an incident report addressing
an issue involving Thomas. Thomas, a 46-year-old African American, is incarcerated for auto theft. Thomas is well known to you because he suffers
from obesity and diabetes mellitus. He receives regular blood sugar analyses
and insulin administration from the nursing staff. In reading through the
incident report you discover that Thomas has been found hoarding the fruit
from his special diabetic diet plate and giving it to fellow inmates. The inmates, it was discovered, were placing the fruit in a container in their cell,
allowing it to ferment, and making alcohol. The alcohol was then used to
barter for items from other inmates.

Although many inmates were involved in this infraction, Thomas was
singled out for punishment because he was the only one known to be involved. He was implicated because of the fact that the fruit used for fer-
mentation is readily available only to diabetics, and Thomas is the only one
on his cell block with access to the fruit.

Thomas has refused to implicate others involved in this incident. He
has been informed by the jail staff that he is at risk for an increased sentence because of his apparent involvement. The jail administrator has informed you that you may be required to "find another way" to assist
Thomas in meeting his special nutritional needs.

When Thomas presents in your office today for his insulin administration, you have a discussion with him about the events of the previous day.
You tell him that you are concerned about his situation, particularly since
the fact that he has been giving other inmates part of his prescribed meal
indicates that he had not been adhering to the strict diabetic diet guidelines.
You inform him that you are not concerned with the legality of his actions,
but you are concerned about the effects they may have on his health and
well-being.

Thomas appears distraught. He tells you, in confidence, that he was
forced by the other inmates to "give them what they needed for their
booze." He adds, "I can't squeal or I'm a dead man." You stress the issue of
patient confidentiality and advise Thomas that you have no influence over
the legal matters of the system, that your job is to help him to get what he
needs to limit the negative effects of the diabetes. You advise him that this
may be difficult given the proposed restrictions on his diet. You decide to
work together with Thomas to identify methods of ensuring appropriate
nutrition for his medical condition while attempting to limit his vulnerabil-
ity to other inmates.

Questions

1) What factors are influencing the way in which Thomas's dietary needs are met?

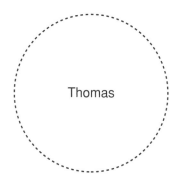

2) In the open system of the jail, what variables can you as the community health nurse manipulate to effect positive change on behalf of, and in conjunction with, this client?

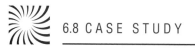

6.8 CASE STUDY

MEDICAL-SURGICAL: BENIGN PROSTATIC HYPERTROPHY AND ELDER ABUSE

SCENARIO

You are a public health nurse working for the adult protective services division of the Brownsville social services agency. You are following up on a referral from a medical assistant who is the office manager for a local urologist. In the referral, the medical assistant expressed concern about the

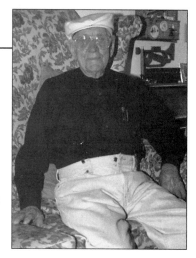

home environment of Mr. Joad, aged 82, who is being followed by the urologist for treatment of benign prostatic hypertrophy.

The medical assistant reports that Mr. Joad is seen on a monthly basis in the physician's office. She states that she has become increasingly concerned about Mr. Joad's safety and well-being based on what she has observed during his office visits over the past 7 months. Specific information related in the medical assistant's report to adult protective services includes the following:

- Mr. Joad has experienced a loss of 12% of his body weight over the past 7 months. His physician reports that there is no apparent disease process leading to the weight loss.
- Reports of statements made by Mr. Joad about the lack of food in his home "because my grandkid keeps taking my Social Security."
- Poor hygiene as evidenced by soiled clothing, matted hair, and frequent fungal infections of fingernails and toenails.

The medical assistant reports that Mr. Joad is dropped off at the physician's office by his grandson, who waits in the parking lot during the visit. She adds that Mr. Joad expresses anger about his living situation, citing statements such as "they don't take care of me . . . they just let me live with them so they can get my checks" but adds "I don't have nowhere else to go . . . and I ain't goin' to no damn home . . . I'd shoot myself in the head before I'd go to one of them homes."

The Joads have no telephone so you are unable to call and schedule your visit with the family. Based on information from Mr. Joad's medical record, you know that he lives with his 39-year-old grandson, Bob, and his family in the mountains outside of Brownsville. The extended family consists of Bob, Bob's 42-year-old wife Denise, and the couple's five children ranging in age from 2 to 21.

As you prepare for the home visit you review a local map to locate the home. You find that the home is located in an isolated area 20 miles outside of Brownsville, 4 miles up a dirt road.

Your goals for the initial visit with this family are to follow up on the report made to your agency and to assess Mr. Joad's physical, emotional, and financial status. You will attempt to determine the risk status and identify the need for further follow-up.

As you approach the Joad's home you note that it is an older cabin-style structure in disrepair. You are met at the door by Denise, who asks "Who in the hell are you . . . what do you want with us?" When you explain that you are a representative of the county's social service agency and would like to talk with Mr. Joad and the family about Mr. Joad's health, Denise allows you to enter the home and instructs you to sit on a couch in the front room. You advise Denise that you would like to speak with the family and then with Mr. Joad privately. She calls for Mr. Joad and Bob to join you in the front room. As you wait for the two men, Denise tells you "I know you're here because he's getting so skinny but he won't wear his dentures . . . we try to make him but he just won't take care of himself."

When Mr. Joad, Denise, and Bob are present, sitting in the front room, you again state your role and the reason for the visit. You are met with stares from Bob and Denise. Mr. Joad's gaze is fixed on the front door.

Questions

1) How do you begin to assess the structure of this family system?
   - What type of questions will you ask at this juncture?

2) Prioritize the issues to be addressed with the family unit. How in-depth do you need to be in your questioning at this point?

3) Discuss techniques that you might use to encourage self-disclosure in a situation that appears to be threatening to this family unit.

4) What positive factors can you identify that you will build on in your relationship with this family system?

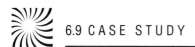 6.9 CASE STUDY

EFFECTS ON CAREGIVER: CEREBRAL PALSY AND CHRONIC OBSTRUCTIVE PULMONARY DISEASE

Discuss potential effects on the primary caregiver of individuals in scenarios A and B.

SCENARIO A

Mary Ann is a 4-year-old girl with cerebral palsy. Her diagnoses include spasticity, significant vision loss, seizures, and developmental delay. Daily care of Mary Ann requires tube feedings, insertion of contact lenses, diapering, monitoring of intake and output, administration of seven to ten prescription medications and provision of prescribed (ketogenic) diet for seizure control. Mary Ann's mother, Jody, is a single mother and Mary Ann's primary caretaker. Jody also has a 10-year-old son.

Potential effects on Jody include:

SCENARIO B

Tom is a 58-year-old man with chronic obstructive pulmonary disease. He is oxygen dependent and suffers from sleep apnea. Tom has cataracts that may require surgery. He takes six prescribed medications per day. Tom continues to smoke and has stated, "What's the difference, I'm going to die anyway." Tom's primary caregiver is his 30-year-old son, Mike. Mike is a long-haul truck driver. He has made the following statements regarding his role in caring for his father. "I worry about him when I'm gone for long periods of time . . . he doesn't eat right and I'm afraid he'll forget to turn off his oxygen when he smokes. I always ask him to turn off his oxygen and go outside when he smokes around me."

Potential effects on Mike include:

References

Spradley, B. W., & Allender, J. A. (1996). *Community health nursing concepts and practice* (4th ed.). Philadelphia: Lippincott-Raven Publishers.

Wolf, G., Boland, S., & Aukerman, M. (1994). A transformational model for the practice of professional nursing, Part 1: The model. *Journal of Nursing Administration, 24*(4) 51–57.

CHAPTER 7

Community as Client

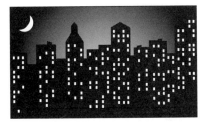

One of the major differences between hospital- and community-based nursing practice has been the identified client. Historically, nurses working in the hospital have provided services to individual clients. In contrast, community health nursing services have focused on individuals, families, aggregates, and communities. Changes in the nursing profession, along with changes in the health care system, have created an environment in which nurses in all settings must consider the community their client. Chapter 7 presents a review of nursing activities addressing the community as the identified client.

REVIEW _____

I. Definitions
   A. Community: The defining characteristics of a community are:
      1. Geographic location
      2. Time period
      3. Shared characteristics/beliefs

B. Client: As a community health nurse, your identified client may be one or more of the following:
   1. Individual
   2. Family
   3. Group
   4. Subpopulation
   5. Population
   6. Community (Spradley, 1996, p. 191)
C. Aggregate: This word is synonymous with population.
II. Application of the nursing process to clients in the community
   A. Health planning model
III. Community assessment
   A. Identification of community characteristics
      1. Population
      2. Location
      3. Social system
   B. Health indicators of the community
IV. Community health diagnosis
V. Empowering communities
VI. Community resources

DISCUSSION

I. Community assessment parameters. The following parameters will provide the community health nurse with important assessment data:
   A. Population
      1. Demographics
         a) Ethnicity
         b) Languages spoken
      2. Numbers
      3. Density
      4. Cycles
   B. Geography
      1. Climate
      2. Physical features
   C. Health indicators
      1. Morbidity
         a) Rates and etiologies
      2. Mortality
         a) Rates and etiologies
      3. Birth rates
         a) Prenatal care utilization
         b) Parental demographics
   D. Environment
      1. Air

2. Food
3. Housing
   a) Homelessness
   b) Cost and availability
4. Water
5. Waste
   a) Hazardous waste sources

E. Industry
   1. Employment
      a) Wages
      b) Stability
   2. Health issues
      a) Exposure to potentially harmful substances
         (1) Pollutants
         (2) Stress
   3. Insurance

F. Education
   1. Value of education
   2. Schools
      a) Class size
      b) Availability of appropriate teachers
      c) Multilingual and multicultural curriculums
      d) Location
         (1) Accessibility
         (2) Transportation
   3. Special education
   4. Vocational training
   5. Pregnant and parenting teens
   6. Parental involvement
   7. Mores (ie, sex education)
   8. Health programs
      a) Education
      b) School nurses
      c) Clinics
   9. Nutritional programs
   10. Junior colleges
   11. Colleges and universities
      a) Cost

G. Social issues
   1. Crime statistics
   2. Unemployment
   3. Gangs
   4. Drug usage (including alcohol)
      a) Demographics of drug-using population
      b) Types of drugs prevalent

   H. Leisure and recreational activities
      1. Community centers
      2. Youth programs
         a) Sports
         b) Arts
      3. Playgrounds
         a) 'Turf' issues
      4. Libraries
      5. Cost and accessibility of programs
         a) Free or low cost (ie, mobile "bookmobile")
         b) Handicapped accessibility
      6. Private facilities
      7. Funding for programs and facilities
   I. Transportation
      1. Public
         a) Buses
         b) Other
      2. Cost
      3. Local or long distance
      4. Handicapped accessibility
      5. Bicycle and walking trails
      6. Private
         a) Taxis
   J. Medical services
      1. Emergency medical services
      2. Accessibility
      3. Clinics
      4. Hospitals
         a) Community
         b) Research
      5. Health care professionals
         a) Availability of appropriate professionals
            (1) Education and training
            (2) Language ability
            (3) Cultural sensitivity
   K. Communication
      1. Local, city, county, state, national
      2. Ownership of media
      3. Television
      4. Newspapers
      5. Radio
      6. Telephones
      7. Computer
   L. Religion
      1. Places of worship

2. Types of religious practice
   a) Judeo-Christian
   b) Jewish
   c) Buddhist
3. Influence of religion on community
4. Acceptance of alternative religions
5. Health beliefs and practices of religions
6. Political involvement and power of religious community

M. Politics
   1. Organization
      a) Districts
   2. Funding sources
   3. Voting habits
      a) Registration
         (1) Methods
      b) Percentage of population voting

N. Public services
   1. Police
   2. Fire
   3. Utilities
      a) Cost
   4. Programs for low income

O. Community emergency response plans
   1. Red Cross (Swanson & Albrecht, 1993, pp. 86–87)

II. Examples of community health resources
   A. Community clinics
      1. Women's clinics
      2. Culturally focused clinics
   B. Dental care
   C. Family planning
      1. Abortion
   D. Pregnancy
      1. Prenatal care
      2. Postpartum care
         a) Doulas
         b) Breast-feeding support
            (1) La Leche League
   E. Human immunodeficiency virus/acquired immunodeficiency syndrome (HIV/AIDS)
      1. Antibody testing
      2. Case management
   F. Services for the disabled
      1. Rehabilitation
      2. Independent living
      3. Service organizations

    4. Easter Seals

    5. March of Dimes

    6. Lions Club

    7. Red Cross

    8. Disease-specific organizations

G. Alcohol and other drugs

    1. Diversion

    2. Treatment

      a) Outpatient

      b) Live-in

    3. Hotlines

    4. Methadone programs

    5. Support groups

      a) Alcoholics Anonymous (AA)

      b) Narcotics Anonymous (NA)

      c) Nicotine Anonymous

H. Community organizations

 I. Hospitals

    1. Programs

      a) Rehabilitation

      b) Restorative care

 J. Home health care

K. Hospice

L. Caregiver services

M. Child health

N. Immunization

O. Maternal and child health

P. Senior health

Q. Mental health

R. Public health

S. County managed care systems

T. Medicaid/Medicare care

U. Nutritional services

    1. Food stamps

    2. WIC: women, infants, and children

      a) Nutritional education and vouchers for food for pregnant breast-feeding and postpartum women. Children up to 5 years of age are served, depending on program funding. WIC is a farm subsidy program.

    3. Senior nutrition services

V. Social services

    1. Child care

      a) Licensing

      b) Monitoring

        (1) Immunizations, health practices

    2. Foster care

3. Adoption
   a) Support groups
   b) Community education
   c) Special needs children
4. Youth services
5. Child protection
   a) Child protective services
   b) Child abuse prevention programs
6. Adult protective services
   a) Intervenes for elderly and dependent individuals with issues of neglect and abuse
7. Parenting
   a) Education
   b) Co-op
8. Support groups
   a) Alternative life-styles
   b) Al-Anon
   c) Mothers Against Drunk Driving (MADD)
   d) Disease-specific (ie, for those who are affected by cancer)
9. Housing
   a) Homeless services
      (1) Health care
      (2) Shelters
      (3) Job training
   b) Rental assistance
   c) Emergency housing
   d) Low-income housing
   e) Migrant farming camps
   f) Senior housing
   g) Habitat for Humanity
   h) Independent living environments
   i) Disabled housing
10. Financial assistance
    a) Aid to Families With Dependent Children (AFDC)
       (1) Financial support to families with children under 18 years of age, families must be low income or unemployed
    b) Churches
11. Social service organizations
    a) United Way
    b) Salvation Army
    c) Aggregate-specific services
       (1) Senior networks
       (2) Neighborhood organizations
12. Translation services
13. Transportation
    a) Commuting

      b) Children's transportation
      c) Disabled passenger transportation
      d) Volunteer drivers
        (1) Red Cross
14. Education and training services
15. Preschools
      a) Head Start
16. School districts
      a) Parent–teacher groups
17. Special education
18. School–industry partnerships
19. Alternative schools
      a) Independent study
      b) Parenting teens
20. Adult education
      a) Vocational training
      b) English as a second language
      c) Senior education programs
21. Employment training
      a) Retraining
      b) Veterans' programs
22. Job placement
23. Greater Avenues for Independence (GAIN)
      a) Individualized career counseling, financial assistance for education and child care for families on AFDC
24. Higher education
      a) Junior college
      b) College
      c) University

W. Recreation and leisure
  1. Camps
      a) Gender specific
      b) Age specific
      c) Sports and arts
      d) For the disabled and chronically ill
  2. Youth organizations
      a) Big Brothers and Big Sisters
      b) YMCA and YWCA
      c) Boys Clubs and Girls Clubs
      d) Girl Scouts and Boy Scouts
      e) Camp Fire Girls and Camp Fire Boys
  3. Youth groups with religious affiliations
  4. Services for the disabled
      a) Sports leagues
      b) Special Olympics
  5. Parks and recreation departments

      6. Community centers
      7. Senior social and recreation
      8. Sports programs
      9. Arts programs
    10. Clubs (science, chess, etc)
  X. Legal and safety-related resources
      1. Advocacy groups
      2. Domestic violence
        a) Legal protection
          (1) Restraining orders
        b) Safe housing
        c) Education
        d) Counseling
      3. Legal services
        a) Legal Aid
        b) Divorce
        c) Mediation
      4. Criminal justice
        a) Police departments
        b) Programs
          (1) Neighborhood watch
          (2) Drug abuse prevention
        a) Education in the schools
        c) Sheriff
        d) District attorney
        e) Probation department
        f) Gang intervention
III. Empowerment of communities using the nursing process. Although the terms empowerment and advocacy are discussed in detail in other chapters of this text, their application to the community as a whole bears some discussion. The skills that the community health nurse uses to facilitate empowerment in individuals and families may also be applied to aggregates and communities. Presented below are nursing interventions that will assist the nurse in the empowerment of communities.
  A. Interventions
  B. Assessment
      1. Identify communities' actual and potential problems and strengths.
      2. Identify community resources.
      3. Identify influential members of the community.
        a) Official (ie, political figures)
        b) Unofficial and official (ie, neighborhood leaders)
  C. Statement of identified goals
      1. Based on community consensus
      2. Ensure that all members of the community have a voice in this process.

   D. Planning
     1. Mutually agree on plan of action involving community members.
     2. Emphasize community's strengths and resources and maximize.
     3. Involve community members.
     4. Ensure that plan will result in positive outcome for aggregate/community.
     5. Allow and encourage all members of the community to present ideas aimed at addressing the issue at hand.
   E. Implementation
     1. Maximize utilization of the community's internal and external resources.
     2. Involve community members in the implementation process.
   F. Evaluation
     1. Work with the community to examine whether goals were met.
     2. Identify areas warranting further follow-up.
     3. Plan subsequent steps with a focus on continued community participation.
       a) Theoretical models for community assessment
       b) Neuman's health care systems model

Case Studies and Exercises

Responses to the following case studies and exercises reflect the ability to:

    1. Define techniques for assessing aggregates and communities.
    2. Perform a community assessment.
    3. Identify factors that affect the health of aggregates and communities.
    4. Distinguish between positive, negative, and neutral effects on health status.
    5. Develop an appropriate plan of action for a health problem facing an aggregate or community.
    6. Discuss appropriate use of community resources.
    7. Describe methods of coordination with community agencies.
    8. Analyze the role of the community health nurse in implementing change in aggregates and communities.
    9. Participate in strategies to prioritize the needs of a community.
   10. Evaluate the effects of community health nursing intervention with aggregates and communities.

7.1 EXERCISE

COMMUNITY

Consider the community in which you reside.

1) Identify five potential stressors to the elderly population in your community.

2) What influence might these stressors have on this aggregate?

3) How might the community health nurse go about influencing:
   • The stressors

   • The aggregate's response to the stressors

7.2 EXERCISE

SUBSTANCE ABUSE PREVENTION

How might a public health nurse working in a health education program of the local health department intervene to decrease the incidence of substance abuse with the aggregate in the following situation:

Prevention of crack cocaine use among 14- to 17-year-olds in Brownsville. The aggregate has been identified by the local police department. According to the authorities, the group has the following characteristics:

• A group of 8 to 10 teens with high truancy and school drop-out rate
• The group "hangs out" during the day at the apartment of a 23-year-old suspected drug dealer.
• Attempts aimed at penalizing the parents have been unsuccessful in changing behavior among the teens.
• The group is suspected in several incidents of violence against local youths from different cliques.

Brainstorm and present your ideas for community health nursing intervention.

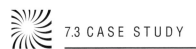 **7.3 CASE STUDY**

HEALTH FAIR

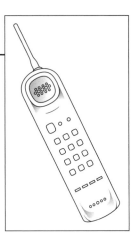

SCENARIO

You are an occupational health nurse working for a large manufacturing firm in Capitol City. Your company produces components for telephone systems. You are planning a health fair that will take place in 3 months. The management staff has informed you that they would like the following issues addressed at the health fair:

- Stress reduction
- Decreased incidence of repetitive motion injuries such as carpal tunnel syndrome
- Reduction in sick time

Question

The management has advised you of their requests for the health fair.

1) How will you go about identifying the needs of your target population, the labor force?

7.4 EXERCISE

ENVIRONMENTAL INFLUENCES ON PHYSICAL AND MENTAL HEALTH

What positive or negative effects might the following have on the physical and mental health of individuals, families, and aggregates in your community:

Factors	Individual	Families	Aggregates
Poverty			
Homelessness			

(continued)

Factors	Individual	Families	Aggregates
Drug and alcohol abuse			
High cost of living			
Low literacy			
Television			
Overcrowded public schools			
Increasing gang activity			
Increased awareness of AIDS			
Boys and girls clubs			
Immunizations			
School lunch programs			

Questions

1) As you formulated your responses, in what ways did you envision nurses in your community affecting these issues?

2) Review your responses and identify specific areas of practice for nurses working to effect change in communities.

7.5 EXERCISE

DATA COLLECTION FOR VARIOUS AGGREGATES

SCENARIO

Following is a presentation of information related to three aggregates living in the Metropolis area.

Area 1

A small neighborhood, four blocks long and six blocks wide located in downtown Metropolis. This urban area is populated by a large number of Vietnamese immigrants, primarily first and second generation. Many of the individuals in this community come from the same geographic area in Vietnam. The primary language of this population is Hmong. The majority of these immigrants have legal residence in this country. Many are attempting to bring additional family members from Vietnam to join them. The unemployment rate in this community is quite low and the major employers are small, family-owned local businesses.

Area 2

An affluent, gated community on the outskirts of Metropolis. This community has 24-hour security service, private road, private schools, a small convenience store, and extensive recreational facilities. The average household income in this community is over $250,000 per year. There is an ethnic mix in this population. Several families living in the community are temporary residents from Germany, many of whom have come to work in the computer industry.

Area 3

This is a large area located in the industrial section of Metropolis, with many older, run down houses and apartment complexes. The children in this area are bused to various school districts because there is no local school. There is a diverse ethnic population. The median age of this population is older than that of the greater Metropolis area. There are several small convenient stores and many liquor stores and bars. The crime rate in this area is high and there are reports of increasing gang activity.

Identify possible resources for obtaining information on the following categories for areas 1, 2, and 3:

Indicators	Area 1	Area 2	Area 3
Crime statistics			
Nutritional status			
Employment stress			
Exposure to hazar-dous materials			
Cultural beliefs about health			
Recreational facilities			
Air quality			
Housing costs and availability			
Special education services			
Preventative health services			
Transportation services			
Gang activity			
School dropout rate			

7.6 EXERCISE

COMMUNITY RESOURCES IN YOUR COMMUNITY

Identify free or low-cost resources in your community for the following:

- Health care

- Dental care

- Nutritional assistance
    Food

    Nutritional counseling

- Financial assistance

- Housing

    Homelessness

- Clothing

- Transportation

- Child care

- Parenting

- Stress management

- Family counseling

- Domestic violence
    Counseling
        Women

        Men

    Emergency shelter

- Teen Pregnancy

- Education
     GED

     Health education

- Services for the elderly
     Elder day care programs

- Caregiver support

1. What sources of information did you use to assist you in this exercise?

     - What difficulties did you experience in obtaining this information?

2. How would you go about gathering additional information related to resources in your community?

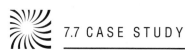 7.7 CASE STUDY

POLICY ON NEEDLE EXCHANGE AND AIDS PREVENTION

SCENARIO

You are a public health nurse working in the AIDS program of the health department in Capitol City. Your community has a large heroin-using population. You have identified an increase in clients with significant risk behaviors presenting to your department for HIV antibody testing. You have been reading public health literature that addresses the issue of local needle exchange programs. These programs offer confidential services, which allow individuals to discard used intravenous drug "works" and receive new, sterile needles and syringes. The literature states that these programs do not increase the

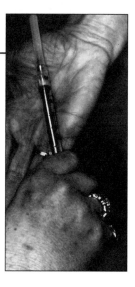

use of illicit drugs. Compelling evidence also indicates that such programs may dramatically reduce the transmission of HIV because there is less likelihood of sharing used "works."

Questions

1) Consider the mission statement of public health. What is your responsibility based on the mission statement and your position within the health department?

2) What actions do you believe are in the best interest of the population of Capitol City?

3) Who must you involve in actions aimed at addressing this issue?

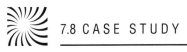 7.8 CASE STUDY

SCHOOLS AND VIOLENCE

SCENARIO

You are a school nurse working in a junior high school (grades 6–8) in Metropolis. You have been asked to participate on a task force working on the development of an after school program for 150 to 200 students whose parents are unable to pick them up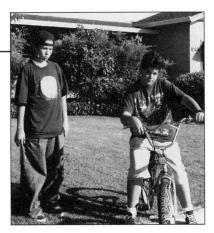
until 5:30 PM. The school day ends at 2:50 PM. The goal of this program is to keep "latch key" children off of the streets. The issue of "latch key" children has been highlighted in the local press in recent months after an accidental shooting in the home of one of the children from this school. The incident occurred when two 12-year-old boys were home alone, playing with a rifle. One of the boys accidentally shot and killed the other.

The program is the brainchild of the mayor of Metropolis. If successful, this program will be a model for other schools in the area.

The task force has been in existence for several months and has already held three meetings. You will be the only nurse on the committee. As a community health nurse, you want to ensure that your perspective is presented and that you are influential in the development of this program.

Questions

1) Who is the aggregate being served in this scenario?
    - Students?

    - Parents?

    - School faculty?

    - Community?

    Explain your response.

2) What questions will you ask about the type of data gathered related to the proposed program? What questions must be answered to ensure appropriate planning?

3) The task force consists of the following members:
    - Mayor's assistant
    - School board president
    - Three faculty members
    - Four members of the parents' association
    - One local business representative (realtor)
    - School nurse (you)

    Are there any other individuals or groups you feel should be represented on this committee? Who?

    Why?

4) The group is having difficulty coming up with options for resources in the following areas; provide them with some ideas.

Resource	Options for Resources
Money	
Staffing	
Volunteers	
Computers	
Exercise equipment	
Mobile services (ie, library, science)	

5) Do you believe that this type of program will benefit the aggregate?

- Do you agree with the mayor, who states that the community as a whole will reap the benefits of this program?

6) Is participation on this task force appropriate in your role as the school nurse? Why or why not?

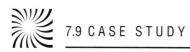 7.9 CASE STUDY

BACK INJURIES

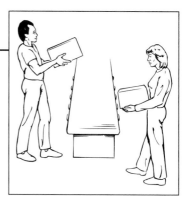

SCENARIO

You have been hired as an occupational nurse consultant by a fruit packing company in Capitol City. The company's insurance rates have escalated because of an inordinate amount of workmen's compensation claims for back injuries. Following is information related to your application of the nursing process in this scenario.

Assessment

Data was gathered pertaining to:

- Agency
  - Training
  - Education
  - Workload
- Production expectations
- Number of injuries
  - Past
  - Current
- Specific information about type of injuries
  - Review of medical records
- Characteristics of injured workers
- Job duties
- Medical conditions
  - Current
  - Preexisting
- Physical condition

An anonymous questionnaire was used to elicit information from management and labor work forces. The only identifying characteristic asked of the respondents was whether they were management or labor employees. The following questions were asked:

- Do you feel that there is a problem with back injuries in this company?
- If so, what do you identify as the problem?
- What do you think is causing the problem?
- How do you think the problem could best be resolved?

Although the results of the questionnaire indicated that both labor and management felt that the company had a problem related to back injuries, it also revealed divergent opinions about the possible causes of this problem. Management employees indicated that they perceived a decrease in productivity in the current work force. They felt that the job and concomitant responsibilities had remained unchanged in the past 5 years but that the work force was unable or unwilling to meet the challenges of the positions. Management respondents cited laziness and incompetence as the factors leading to an increase in work-related injuries.

The labor work force felt that the demands of the job were increasing and that the back injuries were a direct result of this phenomenon. They expressed a desire for less stringent production and packing expectations.

Statement of the Problem

After gathering data related to the topics listed above, you review your findings and develop the following problem statement:

Poor muscle tone and obesity of packing employees, leading to improper lifting techniques, resulting in a 23% increase in lumbosacral strain among packing staff.

Your analysis of the etiology of the problem was different from that of cannery employees. You based your conclusion on statistical and medical data. Although the input of the employees was contradictory, it is relevant because it is a perceived problem and it will be addressed during the planning phase.

Plan

You have several ideas about possible nursing interventions related to this issue. You feel that the issue of increased back injuries would best be addressed with a multifaceted intervention that will focus on musculoskeletal preparedness to meet job requirements.

You realize that you will need participation from various entities to ensure a holistic approach to intervention. You will require the support of management to ensure opportunities for employee involvement as well as consideration of possible alterations in working conditions. Labor employees must be involved in identification of appropriate means of intervention based on the identified problem. The formation of a committee comprised of both management and labor employees will assist in the identification of realistic interventions.

Intervention

Labor and management employees have expressed interest in job training and analysis of workload expectations. Management has agreed to provide work time and company resources to effect the needed changes. Labor employees have agreed to look at personal behaviors and work conditions that may predispose them to back injury.

Questions

IMPLEMENTATION

1) What is your plan, based on the willingness of all involved to participate in your designated nursing intervention?

2) As a consultant, you are contracted to perform six educational sessions. What are your plans for these sessions?

3) What recommendations will you make to company management staff?

4) How will you evaluate your interventions?

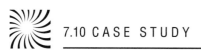 7.10 CASE STUDY

FUNDING DECISIONS

SCENARIO

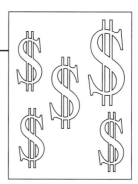

You are a nursing administrator in Metropolis' public health agency. You are presented with the following dilemma:

The funding for county-operated satellite clinics has been reduced by 50% for the upcoming fiscal year. The two clinics in jeopardy are:

1. Sickle cell treatment clinic. This clinic is held monthly in an inner city church. Although the number of clients using clinic resources has decreased slightly in the years since its inception, the clinic is highly regarded by the inner city community and is seen as a sign that "the bureaucracy really can do some good."

2. An HIV prevention clinic that visits several inpatient drug and alcohol rehabilitation programs every 2 weeks. The clinic staff performs

HIV antibody counseling and testing and provides test results and posttest counseling. This program is valued by advocates in the field of substance abuse because it serves a population with high-risk behaviors. It is generally felt that this is a population who might not be tested outside of the environment of the rehabilitation programs.

You will base your decision about elimination or reduction of clinics on assessment data related to each aggregate served by the clinics.

Questions

You will not be asked to make a decision about reducing funding to a particular program. At this point you, as a community health nursing administrator, must have certain information on which you will base your funding decisions. Your responses to the following questions will assist you in the assessment phase of your decision-making process.

1) Who is your client?

2) Who are the aggregates served by these clinics?

3) List identifying characteristics of each aggregate.

4) What are the needs of these groups?

5) Given the information available to you, brainstorm about possible methods of meeting the needs of these aggregates.

6) What criteria would you use to analyze the effects of the eventual funding decision?

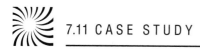 7.11 CASE STUDY

RESEARCH INTO MEDICATION REGIMENS

SCENARIO

You work as a home health nurse in a large home health agency in Metropolis. You specialize in providing home care services for women with gynecologic cancers. Your clients are in various stages of the disease process; some have recently been diagnosed, whereas others are undergoing long-term treatment. Although you serve a variety of clients, your supervisor has begun referring all clients with a diagnosis of uterine cancer to you because she feels that you have developed expertise in this area. You enjoy your work and feel proud of the fact that you are considered by your supervisor and peers to be an expert in this specialty area.

Assessment

Lately you have become concerned about a trend that you perceive to be occurring in many of your clients with gynecologic cancers. Of the 15 clients suffering from gynecologic cancer whom you seen on a regular basis, 9 have expressed significant problems with sleep disturbances, ranging from nightmares and restlessness to insomnia.

You develop a questionnaire to be administered to all of your clients with diagnosed gynecologic cancer. The results of the survey indicate the following relevant assessment data:

- Eleven of the 15 women surveyed reported significant alterations in sleep patterns since being diagnosed with gynecologic cancer.
- Nine of these women are being followed by Dr. Stone, a local oncologist, and six are followed by her partner, Dr. Quinn.
- Ten of the women experiencing sleep disturbances are taking medication XX.

Problem

You deduce that the problems in sleep patterns may be a reaction to medication XX. At this point you will follow up on anecdotal information available to you. Your goal is to identify appropriate steps to be taken at this juncture.

Questions

1) Who is your target population? Is it limited to your home health clients?

2) Who will you involve in the process of planning to address this issue?

3) What input will you need from those involved in the planning process?

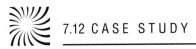 **7.12 CASE STUDY**

PROGRAM DEVELOPMENT FOR DOMESTIC VIOLENCE

SCENARIO

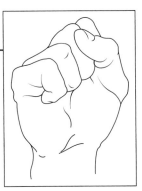

You are a supervising nurse working in a women's health clinic in Smithville. The county Board of Supervisors has approached you expressing concern about domestic violence. They inform you that because there are no services in Smithville for victims of domestic violence, they would like to work with your agency to develop a program addressing this issue.

Historically, clients with issues related to domestic violence, both victims and abusers, have been referred to agencies in Brownsville for services. In recent months, there have been increasing concerns and complaints about the lack of appropriate domestic violence resources available in Smithville.

The interest from the Board of Supervisors comes as a pleasant surprise to you because you and your staff have sought assistance for development of such a program in the past and were unsuccessful in soliciting finding from the Board of Supervisors. Although you feel there is underlying political motivation for their current actions, you will graciously accept their support and assistance.

The Board has offered to provide 'start-up' funding for a program addressing the problem of domestic violence in Smithville. It is their expectation that, if your agency accepts the funding, you will pursue grant funding sources that will provide 'matching' funds within 2 years.

The goals of the program, from the Board of Supervisors' perspective, are:

1. Decrease the incidence of domestic violence in Smithville by 35%.
2. Provide counseling services for victims and batterers.
3. Provide prevention counseling to local organizations.

You would like to see the following issues addressed by the program:

- Outreach to all those at risk
- "Atypical" reportees (ie, men, same-sex partners) for whom the incidence of abuse is significant, but who are often neglected in outreach programs
- Education
  - Women's groups
  - Men's groups
  - Families
  - Schools
  - Emergency response teams (ie, police, fire)
  - Medical professionals
- Institution of a 'safe house' to provide victims with temporary shelter from the abusive environment
- Strict confidentiality among program staff and participants
- Comprehensive data collection methods
- Active pursuit of alternative and additional funding sources

Questions

1) What else would you incorporate into this program?

2) Now that the goals of the Board of Supervisors and your goals have been delineated, how will you assess the needs of the aggregate (individuals affected by domestic violence) related to the issues of:
   - Prevention

   - Education

   - Safety

   - Counseling

3) Discuss methods of evaluating the effects of this program.

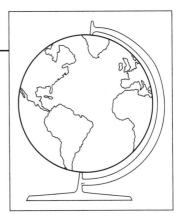

7.13 CASE STUDY

PROGRAM DEVELOPMENT FOR COMMUNITY ASSESSMENT

SCENARIO

As one of the only nurses in your church or synagogue, you have been asked to partici- pate in a volunteer project on an island in the West Indies. Your group has adopted this community as its 'sister city'. The purpose of the 3-week trip is to plan a program that will serve this impoverished island community. You will attempt to identify needs and develop a plan of action that future volunteer efforts will address.

You have the following information about the village:

- Population: 1800
- Medical care: one physician on the island is 17 miles from the village
- Transportation: community taxis (vans)
- Many local 'healers'
- Industry
  - Bananas, coconuts, fishing, emerging tourism
- Languages
  - English and French (most villagers speak at least some English)

Question

1) Discuss the steps you will take in preparing for and performing a com- munity assessment in this situation.

References

Spradley, B. W., & Allender, J. A. (1996). *Community health nursing concepts and practice* (4th ed.). Philadelphia: Lippincott-Raven Publishers.

Swanson, J., & Albrecht, M. (1993). *Community health nursing promoting in health of aggregates*. Philadelphia: Saunders.

CHAPTER 8

Environment of Care

Chapter 8 addresses differences in the provision of nursing care in the community versus the acute care setting. With programs such as postpartum home visitation and cardiac rehabilitation, nurses from acute care settings are extending their practices into the community. The environment of care referred to in this chapter is the community, whether it be the client's home, school, work site, institution (eg, jail) place of worship, or any other community setting. The term 'home' may be used in this chapter to represent any number of community sites, but the focus will be on nurses visiting clients in their homes.

REVIEW

The Home Visit

   I. Assessment of the community
  II. Assessment of the neighborhood
 III. Assessing the home environment
 IV. Introductions
     A. Nurse's position
     B. Agency affiliation
     C. Purpose of visit
   V. Developing rapport
     A. Empathy
  VI. Active listening
     A. Body language
 VII. Use of appropriate questioning techniques for needs assessment

VIII. Identification of problems and strengths
  IX. Identification of mutual goals
   X. Work toward mutually identified goals
       A. Specific assessments
       B. Teaching
       C. Referrals
       D. Role play
       E. Play (with children)
       F. Audiovisual aids
       G. Demonstration and return demonstration
  XI. Plan for future visits
       A. Identify specific tasks for nurse, client, family, and others involved
          in care
       B. Schedule visit date and time
 XII. Documentation
XIII. Appropriate follow-up

DISCUSSION

Planning for the Visit: Safety

Agencies that provide health care services in the community may use a variety of precautions to enhance the safety of their employees. Some agencies send nurses in pairs, others equip employees with personal protection devices such as Mace.® Technologic advances have introduced methods of communication such as cellular phones, which provide added safety for nurses in the community. Although any of these methods may be a reliable means of personal protection, the most valuable assets available to the nurse are constant vigilance and advanced assessment skills. Just as in defensive driving, these skills may alert the nurse to a potentially dangerous situation that may be averted rather than addressed.

Agencies must assume responsibility for providing appropriate safety training to their employees. It is the responsibility of the individual nurse, however, to assess each situation and determine potential threats to safety to oneself and others. A nurse must never enter a situation when, based on this assessment, there is a significant risk to personal safety. Employers must assist employees in defining the degree to which situations are safe or unsafe and must support their employees in taking appropriate safety precautions, such as involving law enforcement, in dangerous situations.

When planning for a visit in the community, it is best to begin by thinking globally. Using the following sequence of questions will assist the nurse in such an approach.

• What do I know about the community?
• What do I know about the neighborhood?

- What do I know about the home or agency in which the visit will occur?
- What do I know about the family unit?
- What do I know about the identified client?
- What additional information must I obtain related to the above and how will I acquire such information?

Preparation

Using a checklist to prepare for home visits will assist the nurse in ensuring readiness. Information that should be included in the community health nurse's checklist is presented below:

  I. Review goals
    A. Agency
      1. Identified problems warranting visit
      2. Expectations of this visit
      3. Number of total visits billable
      4. Length of visits
    B. Community health nursing
      1. Prioritized goals
        a) Mutual nurse/client
        b) Agency
    C. Client
      1. Obtain information about client's goals
        a) From previous visits
        b) From medical record
        c) By contacting client prior to visit
  II. Review client information
    A. Medical status and diagnoses
      1. Review all relevant medical records
      2. Speak with other service providers
    B. Psychosocial status
      1. Support systems
      2. Stressors
 III. Logistics
    A. Location of visit
      1. Travel time
      2. Directions
 IV. Set realistic expectations for visit
    A. Distinguish between long- and short-term client–community health nurse relationship and plan accordingly
      1. Development of trust and rapport
      2. Data collection
  V. Safety
    A. Guidelines
      1. Agency protocol (ie, going in pairs)

  2. Personal
    a) Vigilance (constant vigilance is similar to defensive driving; the nurse must constantly be aware of the surroundings and be prepared to exit at any point if the situation feels unsafe)
    b) Personal protection devices
  3. Vehicle safety (agency or personal vehicle)
    a) Check off safety items before each trip
    b) Use known routes
    c) Park in easily accessible, well-lit areas
    d) Secure vehicle
    e) Ensure easy exit
 B. Technology
  1. Cellular phones
  2. Pagers
 C. Assessing for safety hazards
  1. Community
  2. Neighborhood
  3. Home

Getting in the Door

In the acute care setting, nurses experience little difficulty obtaining physical access to their clients. This is not always the case in community health nursing practice. Although clients may not always welcome the nurse's intervention, there is generally little conflict about roles in the acute care setting. In the community setting, however, clients are on their own 'turf' and experience a greater sense of control over the nurse–client relationship. This phenomenon is an important consideration for nurses working in the community.

Although clients may or may not be invested in the nurse entering their 'turf', a skilled community health nurse has the ability to "sell" himself or herself to clients. This is accomplished by identifying one or more services that the nurse can provide or assist the client in accessing, which the client values. For example, in attempting to set up a visit with a young mother who expresses ambivalence about the services provided by the local health department, the nurse may use as an entrée her knowledge of the WIC program. If the client values the possibility of free nutritional support for herself and her child, she will see value in, and consequently be more accepting of, the nurse's intervention. This process is the first step in mutual goal setting between the nurse and the client as it assists in identification of nursing interventions and community services that are valued by clients.

The process of identifying effective means of enhancing the client's perception of the nurse's services may require a great deal of creativity on the part of the community health nurse. This presents a challenge when working with clients who are ambivalent about services or who may be averse to nursing intervention. Using creativity and consulting with other care providers serving the client will assist in developing appropriate approaches to an individual client. If, however, the client refuses services offered by the nurse, these services must not be thrust on the client.

In the Home: Safety

Safety in the home requires preparation before the visit. Once in the home, the nurse must continue to be vigilant. Assessment of safety in the home will begin on entry, looking for animals and other immediate potential threats to safety. Particularly during initial visits, the nurse must sit in an area that offers an unobstructed path to an exit, should this be necessary. Another consideration for the nurse when entering a client's home is the psychological status of the client, as well as others in the home.

Safety checklists are useful tools that assist the nurse in working with clients to assess and make necessary changes in the home environment. Often these lists are age or diagnosis specific. Agencies should avail themselves of lists designed to address risk-based, aggregate-specific issues.

Sample safety checklist:

- Hazardous materials storage
- Heating and ventilation sources
- Cords (electric, telephone)
- Medication administration
- Medication storage
- Emergency phone numbers
- Locks (including child-proofing)
- Temperature of water heater
- Sources of poison (cleaning solutions, plants, articles containing lead)
- Open water (pools, ponds, toilets)
- Placement of furniture
- Sources of fire
- Potentially dangerous furniture (unsafe bunk beds, bean bag chairs)
- Sleeping position of infants

Adherence to universal precautions is an approach that addresses the safety needs of both the nurse and client. Although the principles remain the same, the application of universal precautions in the home may vary from that in the hospital. Planning for the visit must include identification of all possible equipment necessary for the practice of universal precautions in the home. This equipment may include, but is not limited to, gloves, needle disposal receptacles, and alcohol swabs. The nurse serves as a role model for clients and as such must demonstrate consistency in the use of appropriate techniques.

Assessment of safety in the home will lead to the identification of teaching issues for clients and their families. By identifying positive aspects of home safety, the nurse may begin the interaction with clients on a positive note, for example, "I see that you have a guard around your fireplace; I can see that you are concerned about your child's safety."

Rapport

A common problem for novice home visitors is the tendency to set unrealistic expectations for initial home visits. Although significant problems may be identified when planning for visits, it is important to be realistic about the amount of intervention possible during initial visits. By anticipating that a great deal of time will be spent during initial visits establishing rapport, developing a trusting relationship, and gathering additional assessment data, the nurse may establish realistic goals for these visits. Allowing clients an opportunity for catharsis will eliminate the barrier that exists when clients don't feel that the nurse has a true appreciation for their circumstances.

There is no singular method to the development of a trusting relationship with clients. This is an area that calls on the unique combination of art and science, which defines the nursing profession. The techniques used to develop rapport with clients come easily to some and may prove difficult for others. Similarly, nurses may find that they have difficulty establishing rapport with certain clients and not others.

The establishment of a trusting relationship is the cornerstone of effective interactions with clients in the community setting. If the client is distrustful of the nurse, little change will be effected during the visit. In the absence of rapport, clients are not made to feel that the nurse is genuinely interested in their situation, and they may allow the nurse to dominate the interaction. When the nurse exits the home, however, the reticent client is likely to disregard much of the information the nurse has shared.

Techniques used in the establishment of a trusting relationship include:

- Active listening
- Nonjudgmental response
- Ensuring a clear understanding of roles of client and nurse
- Honest communication
- Expression of genuine interest in clients

Although there may be a specific identified client, it is important to identify and involve other influential individuals in the client's household. If rapport is established only with a singular client, another individual in the home may sabotage the relationship if he or she has not been afforded an opportunity to establish a relationship with and be acknowledged by the nurse.

Assessment

Assessment is the component of the nursing process that varies most significantly in the community versus the acute care setting. This is due to the magnitude of issues that may be present and affecting clients in the environment of care. Although the community health nurse may not address all of the identified issues in his or her interactions with clients, they are all part of the assessment process and must be recognized and acknowledged by the nurse. This means that all assessment data must be considered and then prioritized. Information will be prioritized as:

1. Warranting immediate (possibly legal) follow-up
2. Relevant and significant to the identified problem
3. Identifying a new actual or potential problem
4. A strength
5. A problem warranting referral at some point in the interaction with the client
6. A problem that will not be dealt with in the interactions with this client
7. Inconsequential

Figure 8-1 depicts Maslow's theory regarding the Hierarchy of Needs (Campbell, 1978, p. 16). It is important to note the difference in issues generally identified and addressed in the acute care setting as compared with those identified and addressed in community setting.

Intervention: Prioritization

The amount of time available for direct contact with clients is limited. Generally, agencies allow sufficient time for performance of predetermined functions. Additionally, clients may have time constraints or limited attention span, particularly if they are not completely invested in the nurse being in the home. For these reasons, the success of the visit is contingent on prioritization of issues to be addressed. The following issues must be addressed in the visit:

- Stated goal (based on previsit plan)
- Outcome expected by funding source
- Issues identified once in the home

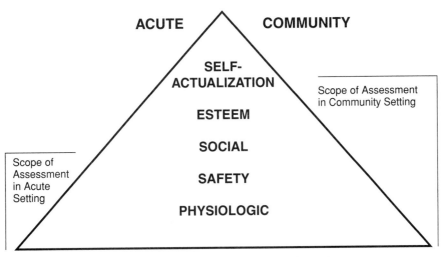

FIGURE 8-1 Scope of assessment: acute versus community setting.

- Client's goals
  - Stated and implied
  - Including those that seem unrelated to the identified problem

DATA RELATED TO NURSING INTERVENTIONS

Nursing literature contains a plethora of information about community health nursing interventions. Home health literature is replete with data regarding the effectiveness of diabetic teaching, dressing changes, and other home health nursing interventions. The future of nursing will present many opportunities for continued research related to the provision of nursing care, particularly highly technical care, in community settings.

Working independently in the community, nurses are making assessments and performing procedures that previously were performed exclusively by highly skilled teams in the acute care setting. Telecommunication allows for the transmission and interpretation of monitoring of physiologic data, such as uterine contractions and cardiac activity, which, until recently, was only possible in the acute care setting. The trend toward early discharge has been accompanied by improved technology in the areas of home infusion, ostomy care, and other nursing specialties.

Although these advances have created new opportunities for community health nurses, there is a concomitant responsibility to keep abreast of new information related to technology and biotechnologic drugs. Nurses must prepare themselves for the expanding role of community health nursing by becoming educated about emerging technologies being used in the home environment.

Setting Limits

Although in some cases nurses experience difficulty gaining access to a client in the environment of care, other nurses are challenged to remove themselves from their interactions with clients. For this reason, the nurse must work toward the establishment of a clear understanding of respective roles between client and caregiver. If accomplished early in the nurse–client relationship, confusion and misinterpretation by either party may be prevented.

Setting limits is accomplished by being clear about roles from the inception of interactions with clients and their families and adhering to professional standards throughout the relationship. This approach may prove difficult, particularly for inexperienced community health nurses, due to the enormity of problems and issues affecting particular clients. The proclivity, particularly for fledgling community health nurses, is either to focus too narrowly (looking solely at the stated purpose of the visit, ie, "I'm here for the decubitus ulcer"), or to become engrossed in the myriad issues facing clients and their families. A skilled nurse is able to identify issues affecting the clients and will work with clients to prioritize these issues and to set reasonable, professional, and mutual expectations for the nurse–client relationship.

Clients with unmet needs may become quite skilled at drawing caregivers in to their problems. This is not necessarily a negative quality because it is a response to unmet needs and may be a type of survival mechanism that demonstrates skills on the part of the client. Faced with these challenging situations, the nurse must become adept at fielding requests and identifying attempts at manipulation. Reinforcing roles and expectations with clients will assist in this process.

Autonomy

Autonomous nursing practice is not unique to the community setting. Although nurses in the acute care setting have traditionally been considered "extensions of the physician," that perception is changing with the emerging definition of the professional nurse. Nurses in all settings are increasingly called on to define their roles and functions in this era of managed care.

Nurses working independently in the environment of care must posses advanced critical thinking skills, self-reliance, creativity, and flexibility. They must anticipate potential problems and situations to be optimally prepared for visits. The community health nurse will be asked to make decisions, frequently without the benefit of immediate consultation with his or her peers.

Extensive knowledge of resources available to the nurse while in the community is critical for successful practice. Should a critical situation, or question that the nurse is unable to answer arise, resources from the employing agency, such as an on-call physician or immediate supervisor, should be available to the nurse. This is especially true because nurses in the community often must respond to situations that would otherwise be addressed by another health care practitioner in the acute care setting.

Follow-up

Coordination with other health care professionals and community resources will occur both during and after the visit. Spending time during the visit teaching clients how to gain access to community resources is an excellent example of effective use of the community health nurse's time. Rather than assuming total responsibility for follow-up, it is important for the nurse to involve the client and the support network in follow-up.

Documentation is another aspect of follow-up and may include an individualized plan of care such as is required by home health agencies, a family chart that may be used by a public health agency, or other method of documentation. Often, documentation used in the community settings varies greatly from that used in acute settings. Agencies must ensure adequate orientation to paperwork, which must include legal aspects of charting, length, and format (such as SOAP).

Conclusion

The autonomous practice of the community health nurse requires advanced critical thinking skills. In most instances, when confronted with an unanticipated or previously unidentified problem, the nurse must make an independent decision about how the issue is to be handled. These skills may be acquired through years of practice in either the acute or the community setting. Critical thinking skills are also being taught in most schools of nursing. Agencies employing community health nurses must work with their staff to ensure an adequate knowledge base related to critical thinking, and must provide ongoing training and opportunity for self-assessment related to these valuable skills.

Case Studies and Exercises

Responses to the following case studies and exercises reflect the ability to:

1. Discuss methods of obtaining relevant assessment data before and during a home visit.
2. List previsit preparation tactics.
3. Report relevant assessment data.
4. Describe appropriate use of screening tools.
5. Identify and prioritize client issues.
6. List strategies for addressing client issues.
7. Outline a plan for a home visit.
8. Explain methods of work with families toward accomplishment of mutual goals.
9. Identify means of evaluating home visits.

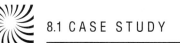 8.1 CASE STUDY

PEDIATRICS: COMMUNICABLE DISEASE—HEAD LICE

SCENARIO

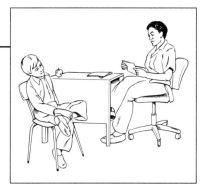

Your client is Arthur Williams, a 9-year-old African American with recurring episodes of pediculosis capitis (head lice); this is his fifth episode. You are the school nurse for Brownsville Elementary School, where Arthur is in the fourth grade. You are responsible for coordination of health services for two elementary and one junior high school. You spend one day each week at Brownsville Elementary School. Protocol for follow-up of head lice is as follows:

1. First episode—informational notice sent to home
2. Second episode—personal notice and phone call
3. Three or more episodes—a home visit

This procedure has been followed in Arthur's case.

Arthur lives with his mother, Ms. Williams, in an apartment complex in Brownsville. Your health clerk spoke with Ms. Williams 3 months ago when Arthur experienced the second episode of head lice. She also lives nearby and has personal knowledge of the family. Based on information obtained from Arthur's teacher you know that Arthur is a bright child who has frequent absences from class. He often comes to school with no lunch and in inappropriate clothing (ie, T-shirts in cold weather). He reportedly informed his teacher that his mother works "a lot" and that he does not know where his father is. He stated that he must stay home to care for younger children when they are ill "since they can't go to day care and my mom has to go to work."

The school health clerk, who has information about this family based on her telephone call, as well as second-hand knowledge of them as members of her neighborhood, informs you that Ms. Williams is a single mother with three children. Arthur is the oldest child; he has a 5-year-old brother and a 3-year-old sister. She tells you that she heard the father was addicted to heroin and that he left town shortly after the birth of the youngest child. Ms. Williams works two jobs. She is employed as a security guard for a manufacturing firm and also works evenings in a local convenience store.

Questions

1) Based on the above information, what are realistic goals for your initial home visit with Ms. Williams and her family?

2) What preparation might assist you in maximizing the effects of you home visit?

3) How will you work with this family to identify mutual goals?

4) What are your professional goals for this family based on the above information?

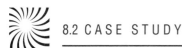

8.2 CASE STUDY

MEDICAL-SURGICAL: EMPLOYEE TRAINING

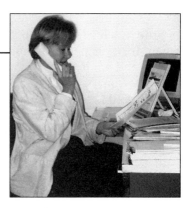

SCENARIO

You are a supervising nurse in a large home
health agency in Capitol City. In discussing
a particular case with a newly hired home
health nurse you identify several potential
problems.

Ms. Saunders is a nurse who was recently hired by your home health
agency. She is a registered nurse with an associate's degree in nursing who
worked in an urgent care center for 3 years after graduation from nursing
school. Ms. Saunders has been with your agency for 5 months.

Ms. Saunders is providing home health services to a family with complex medical and social issues. Her clients, the Mejia family, have been
receiving services from your home health agency for many years. The family consists of Mrs. Mejia, a 41-year-old woman from El Salvador; Mr.
Mejia, a 48-year-old man, also from El Salvador; and their seven children
ranging in age from 4 to 23 years. The youngest child, Ernesto, is the identified client of your agency. Ernesto is a technology-dependent child who
receives regular home health nursing visits for:

- Care of tracheotomy
- Education and assessment related to gastrostomy tube feedings
- Assessment for integumentary breakdown
- Assessment of equipment such as oxygen saturation monitor
- Assessment of parental management of therapeutic regimen
- Fluid, electrolyte, and nutritional assessment

Although Mr. and Mrs. Mejia speak no English, their older children are
fluent in both Spanish and English and are usually available for translation.
Mr. Mejia is employed as a gardener for a local hotel. Mrs. Mejia stays
home to care for the children. She provides most of the care and maintenance for Ernesto and is assisted in these efforts by a certified nursing assistant hired by a local "live at home" foundation. Ernesto's medical expenses
are covered by Medicaid and Medicare.

Recently, Mrs. Mejia has made both formal and informal complaints
that the home health agency "is not doing enough" for her child. She feels
that his condition has not improved as she was told it would and that he
needs more frequent nursing visits than what the family's insurance coverage allows. She would also like the home health agency to provide a nurse
one evening each week so that she and her husband may go out to visit
relatives.

Following a telephone call from Mrs. Mejia, you discuss this case with the family's nurse, Ms. Saunders, who states "I know what's wrong with this family, they just need to make the older kids take more responsibility for the care of Ernesto and they won't do it. Those kids are never home and poor Mrs. Mejia is trying to do everything."

Questions

1) What is significant about the nurse's statement?

2) As her supervisor, what steps will you take to assist the nurse in the identification of mutual goals with this family?

3) What additional assessment data must be obtained by Ms. Saunders?

4) How will you evaluate the outcome of your interaction with Ms. Saunders?

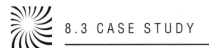 8.3 CASE STUDY

HIGH-RISK INFANT: FOLLOW-UP IN VARIED SOCIOECONOMIC HOUSEHOLDS

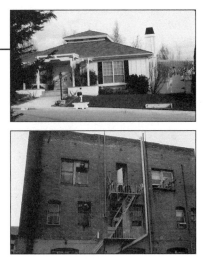

SCENARIO

You are a public health nurse working in the high-risk infant follow-up program in Capitol City. You are responsible for home visits to families whose infants who have been exposed, in utero, to illicit drugs. The determination of perinatal substance abuse may be made prenatally but is primarily identified in routine postpartum toxicology screening. Both of your clients today tested positive for methamphetamines while in the immediate postpartum period.

Mrs. Boyle is your first client of the day; she is a 35-year-old Anglo woman. She lives in an exclusive gated community north of Capitol City. She has private insurance and is employed by a local software company. Her husband is an architect. This is the couple's first child. Prenatal records indicate that this child was the result of artificial insemination. The pregnancy was without complications. No toxicology screen was performed prenatally. When you telephoned Mrs. Boyle to arrange for the visit, she seemed surprised and initially reluctant to agree to the visit. She stated "I know they said there was something wrong with my tests, but I don't do drugs and I'm very upset about their accusations." She agreed to the visit after your assurances that you had information for her about infant development and parenting classes in her community.

Next you will visit Ms. Craig. She is a 21-year-old Anglo woman who lives in a low-income housing complex downtown. Ms. Craig is single and prenatal records indicate involvement by the father of the baby. Ms. Craig's medical costs were covered by Medicaid for this pregnancy. Ms. Craig is gravida three, para one. She has had two therapeutic abortions. Prenatal records document a toxicology screen performed at 7 months' gestation, which was also positive for methamphetamines. At that time Ms. Craig stated that her boyfriend was a "dealer" and that she was cutting down and would eventually attempt to discontinue drug usage. When you telephoned to schedule an appointment for the visit she stated "I know why you're coming . . . it's okay with me but we have to do it when my boyfriend is at work or he'll get mad."

Questions

1) What considerations must be made for safety in preparation for these visits?
   - Mrs. Boyle

   - Ms. Craig

Discuss the following issues as they relate to the initial visit with each client:

2) "Getting in the door"
   - Mrs. Boyle

   - Ms. Craig

3) Establishing a trusting relationship, empathy, and rapport.
   - Mrs. Boyle

   - Ms. Craig

4) Assessing for drug usage
   - Mrs. Boyle

   - Ms. Craig

5) Involving significant family members
   - Mrs. Boyle

   - Ms. Craig

6) Making appropriate referrals
  • Mrs. Boyle

  • Ms. Craig

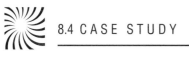 8.4 CASE STUDY

DEVELOPMENT OF RAPPORT— NEW PUBLIC HEALTH NURSE

SCENARIO

This is your first solo home visit in your new role as a public health nurse working for Brownsville County Health Department. After 2 months of orientation, which included observation of home visits, you are excited about the opportunity to perform independent home visits.

Your first client today is Sheila. Sheila is a 19-year-old who has a 3-month-old daughter. Sheila is being followed through the teen parenting program. The goals of this program include:

1. Referrals
   • Support groups
   • Community resources
   • Educational opportunities
   • Child care
   • Employment
2. Education
   • Parenting
   • Birth control
   • Nutrition
3. Assessment
   • Growth and development of the baby
   • Nutritional status of mother and baby
   • Support system

Sheila was recently enrolled in the program and this is her first experience with a public health nurse. You phoned Sheila prior to the visit and reviewed your role and the goals of the program.

When you arrive Sheila greets you at the door and invites you in. She is sitting on the back porch drinking iced tea and smoking cigarettes. The baby is lying in a playpen near Sheila. Sheila tells you that she has been looking forward to your visit. "My friend had a nurse visit her too and she thought it was really cool. I mostly wanted to ask you what I should do about my boyfriend . . . he's such a pain, he isn't helping me out with nothing for the baby."

Role Play

Continue this scenario as a role play with the nurse working to establish rapport with Sheila.

8.5 CASE STUDY

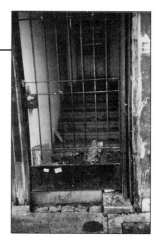

REFERRAL FOLLOW-UP: PARENTING AND NONRESPONSE TO HOME VISIT

SCENARIO

You are a public health nurse working for the Smithville Health Department. You are following up on a referral from a community clinic's family planning clinic. The referral was made for a woman who presented at the clinic and exhibited inappropriate behaviors with her 6-month-old daughter. In their referral, staff stated that they observed the mother shouting at the child, accusing her of "being spoiled rotten." They added that the mother appeared quite anxious and seemed to have difficulty waiting the 15 minutes for her examination. Although the behaviors described in this referral were insufficient to warrant a report to social services, the staff felt that this young mother would benefit from intervention on the part of a public health nurse.

You prepare for this home visit by reviewing the medical records of both the mother and child, making sure to determine if the family has had previous involvement with social service agencies such as child protective services. In addition, you discuss the case with family planning and immunization clinic staff because the family receives services at both clinics. You telephone the client and advise her that you are a nurse with the local health department. You inform her that nurses often visit new mothers to assist them in finding resources. You add that as a public health nurse you will be available to talk with her about her child's growth and development.

The client expresses interest in the visit and states "I want you to show me some things about feeding her and stuff. I need help figuring out what to do at night, she still isn't sleeping much and it's driving me crazy." You advise the client that you will be happy to discuss those issues with her, that you will bring information you will review with her. You add that you noted in her medical record that the father of the baby is living in the home and assure her that she may involve other family members, including the father of the baby, in the home visit. You jointly decide that the visit will occur the next morning at 10:30 and that the father of the baby will be present if his work schedule allows.

On the day of the visit, as you walk up the stairs toward the apartment, you notice someone looking at you through the curtains. As you near the apartment door, the curtains close. Your repeated knocking on the door is met with no response. You call the client's name but there is no answer.

Question

1) Given this scenario, what actions will you take?

 ## 8.6 CASE STUDY

GERONTOLOGY: TRANSIENT ISCHEMIC ATTACKS AND NONRESPONSE TO HOME VISIT

SCENARIO

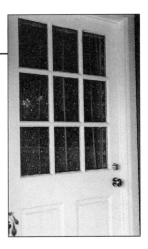

You are a home health nurse in Capitol City. You have been making monthly home visits to Mr. Barker for the past four months. You have a visit scheduled for this morning at 9:00. Mr. Barker is an 82-year-old gentleman who lives alone in a senior citizens' apartment complex. His medical diagnoses include transient ischemic attacks (TIAs) and osteoarthritis. You follow Mr. Barker for monthly assessments of symptoms and medication compliance.

You spoke with Mr. Barker yesterday to remind him of this morning's visit. There is no response this morning to your repeated knocking.

Questions

1) Given this scenario, what actions will you take?

2) How do these actions vary form those taken in Case Study 8.5? Why are they different?

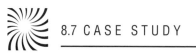 8.7 CASE STUDY

TUBERCULOSIS: CONTACT FOLLOW-UP AND CLIENT RESISTANCE

SCENARIO

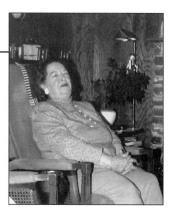

You are a public health nurse working for the health department in Metropolis. You are following up on a family who was seen in tuberculosis (TB) clinic. All members of the family received TB skin tests and four tested positive; all chest x-ray results were negative for TB. It is felt by the staff of TB clinic that the family was exposed to an active case of TB while visiting relatives abroad. The intent of your visit is to assess compliance with anti-TB medications and to inform the family about signs and symptoms indicating drug toxicity.

The family, the O'Malleys, are immigrants from Ireland. The extended family, all who live in the same home, consists of:

- Grandmother O'Malley, a 72-year-old widow who is the matriarch. Twenty-two years ago she emigrated from Ireland with her husband and children.
- Seamus, her 49-year-old son who works as a high school sociology teacher
- Lydia, Seamus' wife, is 47 years old and runs a craft store in Metropolis.
- The couple's children:
  - Sean, 15 years old
  - Patrick, 12 years old
  - Meghan, 8 years old
  - Brittany, 7 years old

Sitting in the home you ask the family about compliance with pre-scribed medications. Grandmother, sitting in the corner of the room, states "I told them not to take those pills, my sister took them and she got cancer . . . those pills are no good."

Questions

1) Following Grandmother O'Malley's statement, what techniques will you use in your attempt to develop rapport with this family? How will you work to enlist the family in the development of mutual goals?

2) What additional information will assist you in achieving this goal? How will you go about obtaining this information?

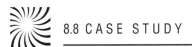 8.8 CASE STUDY

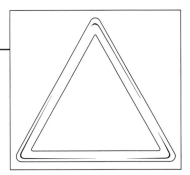

MEDICAL-SURGICAL: MYOCARDIAL INFARCTION

You will be asked to discuss differences in assessment data available to nurses in the roles of cardiac intensive care unit (CICU) staff nurse and home health nurse. Assessment data obtained by these nurses will be presented in excerpts from charting entries in Mr. Marlow's medical record.

SCENARIO

Mr. Marlow is a 61-year-old man who recently suffered an acute myo-cardial infarction (MI). Mr. Marlow was diagnosed with cardiovascular disease at the age of 48 and has been on medication for the treatment of hypertension and hyperlipidemia for the past 11 years. Mr. Marlow's risk factors for cardiovascular disease include obesity (his current weight is 52% greater than ideal body weight), stress (environmental), poor nutrition (diet recall demonstrates an average daily consumption of 42% of calories from fat), and genetic predisposition (both parents died of cardiovascular disease).

Mr. Marlow lives with his wife and two of his children, a 23-year-old son and a 19-year-old daughter. He also has a 28-year-old daughter who is married and lives nearby. The Marlow family lives in a home located in an older neighborhood in Metropolis.

Mr. Marlow works as an accountant for a tax preparation firm in Metropolis. He averages 50 to 60 hours of work per week.

The following excerpts provide information about subjective (S) and objective (O) data obtained by nurses working with Mr. Marlow in the acute and home environments. Nurses' actions (A) are also presented in the excerpts from Mr. Marlow's medical record.

Medical Record
Mr. James Marlow
University Hospital
C.I.C.U.

Admission date: 7/1
Diagnosis: Acute myocardial infarction
          History of cardiovascular disease
Treatment: Angioplasty

Date: Nursing documentation:

7/3   **S:** Family states that they feel pleased with the news from Mr. Marlow's physician regarding his prognosis. "It's much better than we thought it would be," states Mrs. Marlow.
      O: Client is resting comfortably.
      A: See flow sheet for:
          –monitoring: ECG, vital signs, I&O
          –medications: IV, sublingual, p.o.
          –blood drawn for chemistry panel and lipid panel
          –bedrails ^^

7/5   **S:** Patient asking questions about "test results" and prognosis.
      O: Family present with patient. Client awake alert and oriented. Talking with family members.
      A: Discussed with patient and his family:
          –medications being administered, availability of analgesics;
          –plans to transfer to medical–surgical unit;
          –expected date of discharge.
      See flow sheet for:
          –monitoring: ECG, vital signs, I&O;
          –medications: IV, p.o.
          –bedrails ^^
          –instructed patient re:
            turn, cough, and deep breathe
            comfort measures

Medical Record
Mr. James Marlow
University Hospital Home Health Agency

7/3   Initial home visit

S: Client states, "I'm still feeling so tired . . . this diet they've got me on is ridiculous . . . I have no energy . . . can't I change it a little bit, that doctor doesn't know how stressful this has all been . . . I have to keep up my strength." Mrs. Marlow states, "don't worry, I'm going to make him do as the doctor says . . . we can't afford to have him get sick again . . . besides, my daughter and her kids will be coming to stay with us soon so James really needs his strength, I can't be expected to take care of everyone."

O: Three-bedroom home in quiet neighborhood. Home is clean but cluttered. Many piles of clothing and newspapers lying about. Two small dogs and three cats in home. Home is dark. Muted television on throughout visit. Present in the home today are: Mr. and Mrs. Marlow and their two youngest children.

A: Discussed with family:
    −concerns about prescribed diet
        reviewed their understanding of physician's orders and availability of
        University Hospital's nutritionist
    −medication regimen
        signs and symptoms warranting follow-up
        compliance with medication schedule
        planning ahead for refills
    −exercise program at cardiac rehabilitation center to begin in 2 days
    −altered family processes
        ie: daughter with children moving into family home
    −asked family about questions or concerns
    −requested client to keep strict record of diet along with comments about
     dislikes and difficulties related to diet
    −planned for home visit in three days to discuss:
        nutrition
        activity progression
        medications
        fears, anxiety, and stress

A: Nursing actions/interventions:
    −vital signs
    −cardiac and pulmonary assessments
    −assess fluid and electrolyte balance
    −assess activity tolerance
    −discuss self-care activities

7/12   Client home alone
    S: "My wife is at my daughter's house, they're packing up her stuff to move her and her kids in with us." "I've gone off of the diet, I wrote that stuff down for you, but it's been too hectic around here for my wife to cook all of that special stuff . . . my wife is treating me like an invalid so I've decided to take care of myself . . . besides, she'll be busy taking care of my daughter's kids." "I'm afraid my boss doesn't want me to go back to work, he's hoping that I'll quit . . . I'm the oldest guy there and it's getting to be too much but we need the money and the

(continued)

(Continued)

benefits." "I'm too embarrassed to see my friends, I haven't talked to them since the heart attack . . . it's all because I'm so fat, that's why this all happened."
O: Client sat on front porch with nurse throughout visit.
A: Reviewed diet recall with comments and discussed with client alterations that will meet guidelines while making diet more palatable for the client.
  Physical assessment:
  –vital signs
  –cardiac and pulmonary assessments
  –assessment of integumentary system
Used open-ended questions about stress level, available support system and feelings about recovery.
Discussed stress reduction techniques and utilization of available support systems.
  Worked with client on the identification of mutual goals for recovery related to:
  –weight loss
  –exercise
  –medication compliance

Questions

1) Using Maslow's hierarchy, place assessment data gathered by the nurse in the acute and community setting in the appropriate categories on the following graphic.

ASSESSMENT DATA GATHERED BY

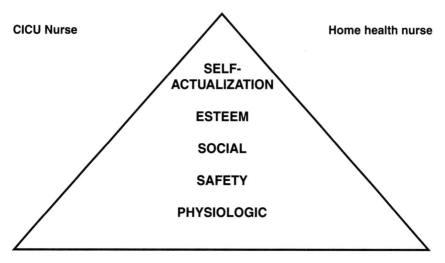

CICU Nurse   **Home health nurse**

SELF-
ACTUALIZATION

ESTEEM

SOCIAL

SAFETY

PHYSIOLOGIC

2) What is the significance of the differences in data available to the nurse in the acute versus community setting?

3) How will you prioritize the issues that you will address with the client and his family in the community setting?

 8.9 CASE STUDY

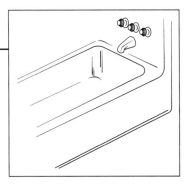

GERONTOLOGY: ALZHEIMER'S DISEASE AND HYPERTENSION

SCENARIO

Ms. Carrol is a 71-year-old woman with stage I Alzheimer's disease (confusion and significant memory loss) and hypertension.
She takes medication for treatment of hypertension and has been on hormone replacement therapy since undergoing a total hysterectomy 7 years ago.

Ms. Carrol lives alone in a large apartment complex in Metropolis. The apartment has two bedrooms, a full bathroom, and a small kitchen. It is located on the third floor of a four-story complex. Ms. Carrol has lived in this apartment for 17 years and has many friends and neighbors who pay her visits on a regular basis.

Ms. Carrol's daily routine consists of:

1. Walking or going to breakfast in the morning
2. Watching the 11:00 AM news
3. Visiting with her in-home helper from 12:00 until 2:00 PM
4. Eating a snack
5. Calling her son at work
6. Walking to a nearby grocery store or visiting with friends in the afternoon
7. Cooking an evening meal

Ms. Carrol's son lives nearby and takes her to breakfast two to three days each week. He has also arranged, and pays for, in-home support service 2 hours each day. Although he values this service immensely, it has become a financial hardship for him to continue to pay his mother's helper.

You work as a nurse practitioner performing routine physical examinations for a medical group in Metropolis. You see Ms. Carrol for follow-up of hypertension and Alzheimer's disease.

Ms. Carrol was diagnosed with stage I Alzheimer's disease 2 years ago. Recently, you have made observations that suggest she may be entering stage II of the disease process. Although Ms. Carrol has been functioning well with the support of her son, her helper, and her friends, you anticipate the need for additional support if she is indeed entering stage II of this disease process.

Questions

1) Identify potential safety risks for Ms. Carrol as she progresses to stage II of Alzheimer's disease.

2) As her primary health care provider, as well as the sole health care professional working in the client's home, how will you prioritize and address these issues?

3) What outcome criteria are appropriate in this situation? How will you evaluate the effectiveness of your interventions?

4) Discuss caregiver role strain as it pertains to this scenario.

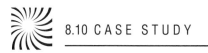 8.10 CASE STUDY

PEDIATRICS: CEREBRAL PALSY

SCENARIO

You are a nurse working with the County Social Service's Foster Care Program in Smithville. Your role is ensuring appropriate medical follow-up for children in the foster care system.

You are working with a family that consists of:

- Lori, a 26-year-old, who is pregnant (23 weeks' gestation) with twins. Lori's physician has prescribed strict bed rest.
- Jim, Lori's partner, a 29-year-old, who is currently incarcerated serving a sentence for possession and sale of crack cocaine.
- Kayla, their 18-month-old daughter. Kayla has mild cerebral palsy with impaired verbal communication and swallowing difficulties. She attends physical and occupational therapy sessions twice each week.

The parents have decided to place Kayla in foster care until after the birth of the twins. Jim's release date is set for 2 months after the expected date of delivery. The fact that the couple has no family members or close friends available to assist in Kayla's care prompted their decision to temporarily place her in foster care.

This is your first visit; Lori and Kayla are present. Today you will review the role of the foster family and will discuss Kayla's medical needs.

The family rents one room in a large home in Smithville. The home is located in a quiet cul-de-sac near Main Street. As you enter the home Lori invites you to sit in the front room. She is resting on the couch and Kayla is lying in a playpen nearby.

You sit in a chair near Lori and begin explaining your role in the foster care system. After approximately 10 minutes, a man enters the kitchen and pours himself a cup of coffee. You glance in his direction and notice that he is glaring at you. You say hello and introduce yourself but he does not respond. He walks toward the front room and sits in a chair between you and the front door.

Questions

1) Are you concerned for your safety? Why or why not?

2) What actions will you take now related to your personal safety?

8.11 CASE STUDY

GERONTOLOGY: COLOSTOMY AND SETTING LIMITS

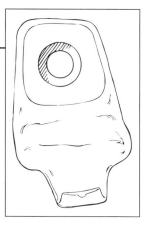

SCENARIO

You are a home health nurse in Smithville. You have been assigned a new client, Tom, an 83-year-old gentleman whose wife of 48 years, Helen, died recently. Tom is receiving home health services for assistance with care and maintenance of a colostomy. Tom has had the colostomy for 5 years, but since Helen's death he has made numerous visits to both his physician's office and the emergency room, with concerns about proper care of the colostomy. Home health nursing services have been approved, as a cost-saving measure, for the purpose of reeducating Tom about self-care of the colostomy.

After introducing yourself to Tom you review the purpose of your visits. You advise him that you will return on two more occasions for the purpose of educating him about his colostomy. Tom seems pleased to have you in his home. He offers you a cup of tea and asks you to sit with him at the kitchen table. "Don't be in such a hurry," he chides you "just take a minute . . . everyone needs to relax once in awhile . . . you're working too hard." During the course of your visit with Tom you find that he seems to have sufficient knowledge to provide self-care for his colostomy. He is able to report signs and symptoms warranting follow-up and demonstrates appropriate aseptic technique in handling of colostomy equipment.

During the visit he asks you to help him interpret an electric bill that he received the previous day. Tom states "I can't understand what they're telling me . . . I'm afraid they're going to shut off my power . . . you have to help me . . . since Helen's been gone I don't have anyone to help me with this stuff." After assisting Tom with the interpretation of his bill, you advise him that it is time for you to go. "Come on," he tells you, "just sit for awhile with a lonely old man . . . you can spare 5 minutes for some more tea."

Questions

1) What issues might be contributing to Tom's behavior?

2) How will you respond to Tom's requests for your time and company?

3) What might you have done to establish a clear understanding of your role?

4) What will you do at this point to clarify your role and time availability?

5) How will you address the issues, such as social isolation, loneliness, and dependency, which seem to be facing Tom?

8.12 EXERCISE

PEDIATRICS: HIGH-RISK INFANT

You are a nurse who worked in the neonatal intensive care unit (NICU) of Capitol City Hospital for 12 years. Your roles included both staff nurse and supervisor. Two years ago, when the hospital underwent major restructuring, you decided that it was time for a change. Along with a colleague, you started an independent nursing practice. Your business has contracts with obstetricians and pediatricians. You provide services such as:

- In-home prenatal monitoring
- In-home infusion therapy (for hyperemesis, etc)
- Postpartum home visitation
- Newborn examinations and follow-up
- High-risk infant follow-up

SCENARIO

Today you will be visiting the Mayes family. The Mayes' child, Sam, was born at 28 weeks' gestation, weighing 2 pounds 11 ounces, and has been in Capitol City Hospital for the past 9 weeks. Sam is to be discharged from the hospital next week and you have been contracted by his pediatrician to provide one predischarge and three postdischarge visits to the family in their home.

Sam is being sent home on an oxygen saturation monitor due to episodes of apnea experienced during his hospitalization. According to his physician, there are no apparent long-term sequelae resulting from his preterm birth. Sam's current weight is 4 pounds 11 ounces. Family information available from the medical record is as follows:

The Mayes family consists of:

- Joanne, Sam's mother, is a 42-year-old patent attorney. Joanne worked up until a week before Sam's premature birth and returned to work 3 weeks after his birth. She pumped her breasts for a week but discontinued at that time.
- William, Sam's father, is a 45-year-old Japanese American man who is unemployed. William plans to stay home with Sam until the infant reaches 6 months of age. William visits Sam in the hospital for several hours each day and has learned a great deal about his care.

Role Play

Each participant should review his or her role in preparation for the role play.

- Roles
  - Nurse
  - Joanne
  - William

NURSE

You have only one visit before Sam is discharged from the hospital. Although you have a great deal of medical information about Sam, you have little information about psychosocial issues affecting his family.

Based on the information available to you, you anticipate and prepare for the following actual and potential family issues:

- Medical
  - Care of a high-risk newborn
  - Nutritional needs of the newborn
  - Oxygen saturation monitor
- Psychosocial
  - Anxiety
  - Guilt
  - Parental roles
- Other
  - Scheduling (Joanne is working full-time)
- Add any additional issues you would like to address

JOANNE

You and William tried unsuccessfully for many years to conceive a child. You were both elated that, through in vitro fertilization, you became pregnant with Sam. Although you were worried that you were "getting too old," you had taken good care of yourself and felt ready to have a child. When William lost his job as a construction foreman early in the pregnancy, you felt stressed but felt that you could "hold things together" with your job as an attorney.

As the pregnancy progressed, however, you discovered that William was having a difficult time finding employment and that he began discussing the possibility of staying home with the baby "for awhile" after the birth. You became increasingly concerned about the family's financial situation and began working longer hours in hopes of bringing in new clients. You wanted to be financially secure in preparation for the birth of the baby.

When you experienced vaginal bleeding and began having contractions at 27 weeks' gestation, you decided to take the doctor's advice and slow down. The contractions did not stop, however, and you delivered Sam at 28 weeks' gestation.

After your initial shock, you became frightened. You were vacillating between fear that Sam would not survive and anxiety about the prospect of parenting a child with significant health care problems. You did not discuss your concerns with anyone.

As soon as you were physically able, you returned to work, thinking that because you felt useless looking at Sam in the hospital, at least you could help your family by working to ensure financial security.

Now that Sam is coming home you feel pleased that "the doctors say he'll be okay" but you have anxiety related to the care of a newborn because you have not had experience in this area. You also feel anxious about the monitor but feel that William will worry about that because he is more familiar with the technology. You realize that you are feeling both guilt and jealousy about William's relationship with Sam, about the bonding that occurred during the past weeks of Sam's hospitalization, but you have not discussed these issues with William.

You are ambivalent about a nurse coming into your home. Although you welcome the information, you feel that the nurse is going to consider you a bad parent because you have not been present at the hospital and because you are not breast-feeding Sam.

WILLIAM

You are elated at the prospect of bringing your son home. You feel concerned about Joanne. You know that something has been bothering her and you think it may be your desire to stay home with Sam. You feel comfortable with the prospect of caring for Sam at home because you learned a great deal from the nurses in the hospital.

You welcome the nurse's presence and hope that Joanne will "open up" to the nurse and discuss what has been bothering her. You have little interest in learning technical skills from the nurse because you do not see this as a need.

Role Play Activity

Role play the initial home visit with learners assuming the roles of: nurse, mother, and father.

The home visit has been scheduled via a telephone call with William, for 4:00 PM today. Joanne will leave work early to be present.

Initiation and previsit phases of the interaction have already occurred.

Work through the following phases of the home visit:

- Introductions
  - ○ Introduce self and role
  - ○ Establish rapport and relationship with clients (begin with informal discussion)
- Implementation
  - ○ Implementation of nursing activities
  - ○ Collection of data, education, and 'hands on'
- Termination
  - ○ Review visit activities, discuss responsibilities for follow-up activities, and plan subsequent visit with family

 8.13 CASE STUDY

PSYCHIATRIC: CAREGIVER ROLE AND IDENTIFYING GOALS

SCENARIO

You are a home health nurse in Smithville. Today you will begin following a new client, Emmit. Emmit is 50 years old and lives with his 83-year-old mother, Alice, in rural Smithville. Emmit is a veteran of the Vietnam War. His diagnoses include:

- Paranoid schizophrenia with delusions
- Hypertension
- Coronary artery disease (CAD)
- Peripheral neuropathy
- Hypertension

Emmit receives home health nursing services to monitor compliance with medications and to assess complications related to his multiple diagnoses. Since the nearest Veteran's Hospital is located in Capitol City, Emmit's physician determined that home health services would provide the most cost-effective means of ongoing care. Emmit's case is currently under review for possible benefits related to agent orange exposure leading to peripheral neuropathy.

Emmit's daily medication regime includes seven drugs prescribed TD or BID and nitroglycerin prn. He receives home health nursing visits three to four times each week for the purposes of:

- Assessment and education regarding compliance with medications
- Physical assessment, including cardiovascular and pulmonary
- Assessment of mental health status and adequacy of caregiver support
- Follow-up on complaints of fatigability with activities of daily living
- Assessment and referrals regarding caregiver support
- Foot care

Before your initial visit with Emmit, you discuss the case with his previous nurse, James. James informs you that he has provided home health nursing services to Emmit for more than 2 years. He states that Emmit is pleasant but that he frequently exhibits inappropriate behavior and adds "you'd better be ready to deal with it." Primarily, Emmit's behavior focuses on expressing his anger about issues in the news. James reports that Emmit keeps abreast of political and other news events and that he has a propensity to become loud and angry when expressing his views. Emmit also insists that he is capable of living independently. Despite numerous complications due to inappropriate self-medicating, Emmit has stated repeatedly "I don't want any help from anyone, I don't mind you all visiting us, but I can take care of myself and my mother just fine."

James informs you that Alice seemed resistant to his intervention during the first year of the home visitation but that she "came around" eventually. Due to Emmit's inconsistency in self-medicating, Alice has assumed responsibility for administering all medications. She has made formal requests to Emmit's physician and the Veteran's Hospital to receive daily home health visits as well as a live-in support person. In reviewing previous notations in the chart you see that Alice relates an inability to pay "with my pension; besides," she added, "they messed up his mind . . . they should pay to take care of him." She informed James that "if something happens to me they'll just let him die . . . we have no other family to take care of him." She has frequently stated that the responsibility of caring for Emmit "is taking its toll on me."

Given the information available to you, you identify the goals of the involved parties:

- Agency goals: assessment, monitoring, and education of existing medical conditions; caregiver support

- Veteran's hospital and physician goals: maintenance of ongoing care needs in a cost-effective manner
- Caregiver goals: emotional and financial support, increased level of supportive services
- Client goals: increased independence

Questions

1) Based on this information, what are your goals for the initial visit with this family?

2) If you were to approach this situation with the goal of accomplishing all of the agency's goals each visit, what do you anticipate would occur during your initial visit? Why?

3) Conversely, what do you predict the outcome of the visit would be if you attempted to address only the issues that Emmit and Alice felt were important?

4) How will you "sell" yourself and your services in this situation?

5) Prioritize your goals and objectives.
   #1:

   #2:

#3:

#4:

Reference

Campbell, C. (1978). *Nursing diagnosis and intervention in nursing practice*. New York: John Wiley & Sons.

CHAPTER 9

Principles of Public Health

Many of the major issues facing society today are responsive to intervention by the public health system. Problems such as violence, substance abuse, and communicable disease have garnered the attention and concern of the populace. Consequently, nurses working in the public health system are increasingly being asked to address these complex issues. All professional nurses, regardless of practice area, must be familiar with the principles of public health to be able to plan effective nursing interventions for clients in today's world. This chapter presents a review of the concepts of epidemiology and prevention as they relate to the provision of nursing care in the community setting.

REVIEW

Definition

"Public health is the effort organized by society to protect, promote, and restore the people's health, emphasize the prevention of disease and the health needs of the populations as a whole. Public health activities change with changing technology and social values, but the goals remain the same: to reduce the amount of disease, premature death, and disease-produced discomfort and disability" (Sheps, 1976, p. 3).

I. Key concepts of epidemiology: Epidemiology is the scientific backbone of public health practice. It is the study of the determinants and incidence of health and disease. Epidemiologic principles may be applied to communities, aggregates, and individuals.

Epidemiology analyzes the interrelationship among the three variables: host, agent, and environment. When these three factors are in a state of equilibrium, a state of health exists. Imbalance of the epidemiologic triad leads to disease.

A. Host factors
   1. Age
   2. Gender
   3. Genetics
   4. Ethnicity
   5. Psychosocial issues
B. Agent factors
   1. Vector
   2. Bacteria
   3. Virus
   4. Chemicals
   5. Lack of substances
C. Environmental factors
   1. Physical
   2. Biologic
   3. Social
D. Epidemiologic reporting
   1. Reportable diseases
   2. Methods of investigation
   3. Reporting methods
      a) Case rate
      b) Morbidity
      c) Mortality
II. Organization of the public health system
A. Jurisdictions
   1. Federal
   2. State
   3. Local
B. Roles
   1. Health officer
   2. Program administrators
   3. Public health nurses
   4. Other health care professionals

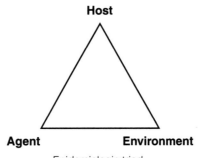

Epidemiologic triad.

III. Preventive health care
    A. Level 1—primary prevention
        1. Prevention of problems before they occur
        2. Health promotion and specific intervention
    B. Level 2—secondary prevention
        1. Early detection, diagnosis, and treatment or intervention
    C. Level 3—tertiary prevention
        1. Limitation of disability, prevention of deterioration
        2. Rehabilitation
IV. Core functions of public health (Feingold, 1984, p. 727)
    A. Surveillance and monitoring
    B. Environmental protection
    C. Disease and injury control
    D. Education
    E. Quality assurance
    F. Laboratory services
    G. Mandated public health services (ie, smoking ordinances, prenatal services)

Application of the Nursing Process— Focus on Public Health

ASSESSMENT

1. What data are available to you?
2. What additional data do you need for a comprehensive assessment?
3. How will you obtain the data?

PROBLEM STATEMENT

1. Identification of
   - Host: who
   - Agent: where and when
   - Environment: why and how
2. Identification of strengths
   - Resources
   - Support system

PLAN

Outcome criteria are mutually developed.

IMPLEMENTATION

1. Levels of prevention
   - Primary: prevent before onset of disease process

- Secondary: early detection and treatment of existing illness
- Tertiary: intervention aimed at reducing the extent and severity of disease

EVALUATION

Evaluation is based on predetermined outcome criteria.

DISCUSSION

Revisions in management of the country's health care system have led to changes in the practice of public health nursing. Health care reform has introduced new variables into the equation of host, agent, and environment. Limited resources and focus on cost containment present benefits as well as new obstacles for the provision of appropriate services to clients. Increased access through county managed care programs may lead to a greater percentage of the population receiving care and thus an overall decrease in morbidity and mortality. Although services will be limited, a larger portion of the community may avail themselves of those services.

In addition, the control of certain communicable diseases, along with the resurgence of others, has led to a shift in focus by public health professionals. Diseases such as acquired immunodeficiency syndrome (AIDS) and tuberculosis (TB) are replacing communicable diseases such as influenza, pneumonia, and diphtheria as major public health concerns. Nurses are identifying new ways of addressing emerging and resurgent health issues. Nursing research is identifying appropriate nursing interventions aimed at combating these problems. Public health nurses have been, and will continue to be, leaders in the pursuit of this type of knowledge.

Societal and technologic changes have also affected public health nursing practice. Technology is now widely available for use in the home. Although public health nurses have traditionally dealt more with the psychosocial aspects of clients' care, there will be increasing need for those nurses to develop skills in direct ('hands on') care of clients, as well as skills in working with new technologies.

It behooves nurses to take advantage of available technology to enhance their practice. The "information age" has allowed nurses to exchange information with clients and colleagues in unprecedented manners. Computers provide opportunities for improved communication. Through the use of technology, such as computer linkage, nurses are developing collegial relationships with other health care professionals as teams communicate and coordinate care of clients.

The vast amount of information necessary to assist in identification of determinants of disease is now readily available with the use of technology. Nurses may use computers to analyze disease prevalence and to identify trends in morbidity and mortality.

Although many societal changes are favorable, some present new problems for the health of communities. Examples of issues that are becoming increasing public health problems in society today include:

- Violence
- Substance abuse
- Diminishing resources
  - Financial
  - Environmental
- Social isolation

Case Studies and Exercises

Responses to the following case studies and exercises reflect the ability to:

1. Differentiate among host, agent, and environmental factors.
2. Distinguish among primary, secondary, and tertiary preventative measures.
3. Relate morbidity and mortality rates to scenarios.
4. Assess for factors that would influence the epidemiologic triad.
5. Provide examples of host, agent, and environmental factors.
6. Develop a plan of primary, secondary, and tertiary interventions.
7. Discuss ways in which specific community health nursing interventions affect the epidemiologic triad.
8. Provide examples of appropriate means of intervening given various client situations.
9. Evaluate the impact of community health nursing interventions.

9.1 EXERCISE

CATEGORIZING HOST, AGENT, AND ENVIRONMENTAL FACTORS

State whether the following factors fall into the category of host, agent, or environment.

Factors	Host	Agent	Environment
Pollution			
Mental illness			
Overcrowded housing			

(continued)

Factors	Host	Agent	Environment
High cholesterol levels			
Salmonella			
HIV			
Immunosuppression			
Heroin			
Age			
Vitamins			
Poverty			
Pregnancy			
Limited food resources			
Ethnicity			
Climate			
Exercise			
Food choices			
Advanced technology			
Genetics			
Bureaucracy			

9.2 EXERCISE

INTERVENTION: PRIMARY, SECONDARY, AND TERTIARY PREVENTION

State ways in which a district public health nurse might intervene with clients to effect positive change, given the following problems. Distinguish among primary, secondary, and tertiary preventive measures.

Public Health Nurse Preventative Interventions

Client Problem	Primary	Secondary	Tertiary
Absence of material attachment			
Mental illness			
High-risk behaviors for HIV infection: multiple partners without use of safer sex practices			
High-risk behaviors for HIV infection: sharing of IV drug "works"			
Inappropriate use of medications among the elderly			

 9.3 CASE STUDY

PEDIATRICS: PLANNING FOR INCREASING IMMUNIZATION RATES

SCENARIO

You are working as a district public health nurse in Capitol City. You are advised by the coordinator of the

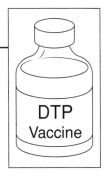

DTP Vaccine

county's immunization program that one of the local neighborhoods has an alarmingly low 38% rate of current immunization for children entering kindergarten.

Demographic Information

The neighborhood in this scenario is located near the freeway in Capitol City. There is a large immigrant population from Pakistan, both documented and undocumented. There is a high poverty rate as well as a large unemployed population. The nearest health department is 6 miles away. There is a bus stop four blocks from the center of the neighborhood. There is a WIC satellite clinic held in a neighborhood mosque every 2 weeks.

Questions

1) Discuss issues that may be contributing to the low rate of immunization among this population.

2) As a public health nurse, how will you respond to this situation. Describe how you will formulate your plan of action; include statements about additional assessment data that will assist in development of your plan.

9.4 EXERCISE

CATEGORIZING PRIMARY, SECONDARY, AND TERTIARY PREVENTION

Identify the levels of prevention in the following examples:

	Primary	*Secondary*	*Tertiary*
Screening of sexually transmitted diseases			
Instruction about safer sex practices			

(continued)

	Primary	Secondary	Tertiary
Teaching about diabetic diet			
Immunizations			
Teaching a family about dental care			
Teaching a client about insulin administration in the home			
Assisting families with housing resources			
Teaching AIDS education in a local high school			
Organizing a health fair			
Working with communities toward removal of hazardous waste			
Teaching parenting skills to parenting high school students			
Working with the Red Cross in a disaster shelter			

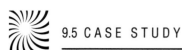 9.5 CASE STUDY

COUNSELING FOR POSITIVE HIV ANTIBODY TEST

SCENARIO

You are a nurse working in a women's jail in Capitol City. You are working with a young woman who has tested positive for human immunodeficiency (HIV) antibodies. She learned her test results 2 months ago. She is scheduled to be released from jail in 2 weeks. She states that she is experiencing increasing anxiety about divulging her test results to her husband.

Your client is Keisha, aged 38, who was incarcerated for possession and sale of heroin. She has a prior arrest record for solicitation and petty theft. Keisha is married and has two sons, ages 4 years and 18 months. Her husband is caring for the children at home because he has been unsuccessful in finding employment. He has been unemployed for over 2 years.

While in jail Keisha has become active in the Narcotics Anonymous (NA) meetings and has spoken with counselors about her drug addiction. Counselors from the local health department performed the HIV antibody testing and discussed Keisha's results with her at length. Keisha has been reluctant to reveal her HIV status to the staff from the jail until today, when she requested a visit with you. She has asked you to help her "get ready" to discuss her test results with her family. She states that she feels that she can trust you to give her "good advice." Keisha would also like to discuss the implications of her test results with you.

Questions

1) How will you counsel Keisha:
   - About discussing her serostatus with her husband

   - About the possible implications of this test result

2) What (if any) mandatory reporting requirements are applicable in this situation?

3) Identify actual and potential host, agent, and environmental factors related to Keisha's HIV antibody status. Include potential past and present modes of transmission.
   - Host

   - Agent

   - Environment

4) How will you discuss methods of prevention of HIV transmission with Keisha?
   - Primary

   - Secondary

   - Tertiary

9.6 EXERCISE

GERIATRICS: NUTRITIONAL DEFICIENCIES

Depression and loneliness are factors that contribute to nutritional deficiencies in the elderly population.

Discuss methods that assist this population in meeting their nutritional needs.

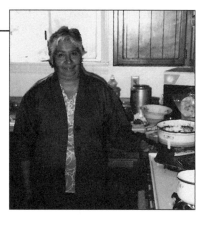

Community Health Nurse Interventions	How Interventions Affect Epi Triad

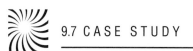

9.7 CASE STUDY

POLICY DEVELOPMENT IN A PRISON ENVIRONMENT

SCENARIO

You have been working as a nurse in a large prison, outside of Metropolis, for 4 years. Recently you were promoted to the role of supervisor. You are now responsible for analysis of health care services for the prison. You look forward to the opportunity to address some of the negative health practices that you have observed in your time as a staff nurse working in the system. You feel strongly that previous supervisors have been remiss in failing to address serious health issues facing the prison population. You plan to implement policies and programs that will address these issues and lead to a healthier environment for the inmates and staff.

The health issues you plan to address include:

- Substance use among inmates
- Noncompliance with medications
- Unsafe sexual practices among inmates

Demographics of prison population:

- Gender: all male inmates and guards
- Number: 700 to 900 inmates on average

Staff:

- Guards are employees of the state correctional department.
- Health care providers are employees of the local health department.
- Health care staff consists of one male physician, one male and one female physician assistant, and four female and two male registered nurses.

The following three case studies present questions related to this scenario.

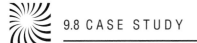 9.8 C A S E   S T U D Y

SUBSTANCE ABUSE AMONG INMATES

SCENARIO

See 9.7 Case Study.

The problem of substance abuse among inmates in the Metropolis prison has been identified and discussed by previous administrators. Attempts have been made to address the issue. Interventions have included group education, counseling by local drug diversion program staff, and weekly Alcoholics Anonymous (AA) and NA meetings. Although some inmates have expressed interest in these approaches, the problem of substance abuse remains rampant.

You have gathered anecdotal information, from health service staff, correctional officers, and inmates, regarding the extent of the problem and believe that the drug-using population in this facility is comprised of a demographically mixed subculture of about 30% of the total population. It is generally believed that the most common drugs being used by prisoners include crack cocaine and heroin. Needles and syringes are valuable commodities and are used in the underground bartering system. It is highly likely that these intravenous drug "works" are being shared by inmates without cleaning between users.

Question

Discuss your application of the nursing process to address the issue presented above. Use information available to you given the scenario, and extrapolate when information is unknown.

ASSESSMENT

1) Epidemiologic triad (list all possible contributing factors)
   - Host factors

   - Agent

   - Environmental factors

2) Problem statement

3) Plan
   - Primary prevention

   - Secondary prevention

- Tertiary prevention

4) Resources available to address issue

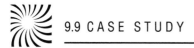 9.9 CASE STUDY

NONCOMPLIANCE WITH MEDICATIONS

See 9.7 Case Study.

SCENARIO

Approximately 3% of the prison population has been prescribed medication for TB prophylaxis. Although compliance with TB medication is high while incarcerated, many of these individuals stop taking the medication immediately after release from prison. Local health department officials have asked for your assistance in this matter. They feel that proper education before release from prison may increase compliance rates after release.

Although you would like to take credit for high compliance level during the period of incarceration, you realize that this is likely because inmates look forward to the personal interaction with nurses, albeit for a brief period of time, when daily medications are administered.

Question

Discuss your application of the nursing process to address the issue presented above. Use information available to you given the scenario, and extrapolate when information is unknown.

ASSESSMENT
1) Epidemiologic triad (list all possible contributing factors)
   - Host factors

- Agent

- Environmental factors

2) Problem statement

3) Plan
  - Primary prevention

  - Secondary prevention

  - Tertiary prevention

4) Available resources

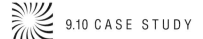 9.10 CASE STUDY

UNSAFE SEXUAL PRACTICES

See 9.7 Case Study.

SCENARIO

You feel strongly that previous supervisors, as well as health department management staff, have long ignored the issue of unsafe sexual practices among inmates. This is an emotionally charged issue that few people have been willing to address. Now that you are responsible for examining the health issues affecting the incarcerated population, you will assume the challenge of beginning to investigate the extent and ramifications of this problem.

You have limited, primarily anecdotal, information about the problem of unsafe sexual practices among inmates. You have learned that:

- Sexual acts are used in the underground bartering system.
- Sexually transmitted diseases often go untreated during the period of incarceration.
- Nonconsensual sex (rape) occurs frequently yet is rarely reported to staff.
- One inmate informed you that by his estimation more than 30% of inmates are practicing unsafe sex.
- Condoms are not available to inmates.
- Previous attempts to make condoms available to inmates were unsuccessful. The Department of Corrections felt that the provision of condoms would condone illegal activities in the jail such as sodomy and transporting of drugs (condoms are often used to smuggle drugs).

Question

Discuss your application of the nursing process to address the issue presented above. Use information available to you given the scenario, and extrapolate when information is unknown.

ASSESSMENT
1) Epidemiologic triad (list all possible contributing factors)
   - Host factors

- Agent

- Environmental factors

2) Problem statement

3) Plan
   - Primary prevention

   - Secondary prevention

   - Tertiary prevention

4) Available resources

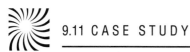 9.11 C A S E   S T U D Y

PEDIATRICS: RESEARCH ON ACUTE LYMPHOID LEUKEMIA

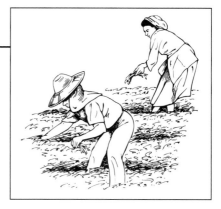

SCENARIO

You are a district nurse working for the health department in Brownsville. The nursing director of Metropolis Hospital has asked to come and speak with the health department staff who provide services to the families living in a large migrant farm worker camp located outside of Brownsville. She informs you that her staff has noticed a disproportionate number of children, who reside in the camp, presenting for care at her facility with the diagnosis of acute lymphoid leukemia (ALL). Although this information is purely anecdotal, she has requested further investigation by public health nurses serving the population in question. Her goal is to obtain sufficient preliminary assessment data to request a formal investigation of the problem by the Centers for Disease Control and Prevention (CDC).

You request 'special assignment' duty to research the problem, realizing that you will need to gather additional data related to morbidity and mortality. The following assessment data are available to you:

- The migrant farm labor camp has 46 residential units.
    - It is owned by the local growers' association.
    - Rent is $400 a month for a two-bedroom unit.
    - The camp has a history of problems related to rent gouging and rodent infestation.
- The population of the camp is fairly stable.
    - Many homes are shared by two or more families.
    - Many families are undocumented workers from Mexico and El Salvador.
    - Most families are two-parent families, first generation immigrants.
- Workers pick strawberries in the summer and apples in the fall.
    - Off-season workers often work in local nurseries.
    - Wages are low and many workers are paid 'under the table.'

To research the issue of possible high rates of ALL among this population, you must first identify the extent of the problem.

Questions

1) Discuss methods of obtaining the following information:
   - Morbidity and mortality of ALL
     - In the general population

     - In the target population

   - Discuss methods of quantifying the variance in rates

2) Given the information available to you, discuss potential influencing factors related to:
   - Host

   - Agent

   - Environment

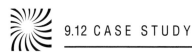

9.12 CASE STUDY

GERONTOLOGY: STAFF EDUCATION

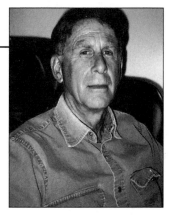

SCENARIO

Sunny Acres is a skilled nursing facility with 49 beds. The staffing pattern for the agency is as follows:

- One registered nurse per shift
- One licensed vocational nurse (LVN) for every eight clients
- One medical assistant for every two LVNs

The facility is part of a group of homes owned and operated by three retired dentists.

Clients range in age from 42 to 98 and have varied psychological and medical problems. Common medical conditions affecting clients include:

- Chronic obstructive pulmonary disease
- Congestive heart failure
- Organic brain syndrome and dementia
- Peripheral neuropathy
- Osteoporosis
- Postcerebrovascular accident
- Depression

There are 49 residents at Sunny Acres. Eighty percent of the residents of Sunny Acres have Medicare as their sole means of payment. Fifteen percent have Medicare and Medicaid and 5% are private-pay clients.

Sunny Acres is located in Smithville and offers the following services to its clients:

- Three meals per day
- Nutritionist consults once every 2 weeks
- Social hour (singing, etc) 9 to 10 AM and 3 to 4 PM
- Physical and occupational therapy weekly
- Assistance with activities of daily living including feeding and bathing
- Administration of medications
- Volunteers daily (ie, animals brought by local animal shelter volunteers, drama productions by local elementary schools)

In your role as the program manager supervising the adult health programs for the local health department, you have been approached by several family members of the residents of Sunny Acres. The families have become concerned about what they perceive to be inadequate provision of basic hygiene services to the clients at Sunny Acres. As examples, they cite instances of ingrown toenails, dirty and overgrown fingernails, dermatitis of the scalp, and scabies. They report having sought assistance from the owners, to no avail.

They have been advised by the operators of the facility that if they would like additional services for their family members, they will be required to provide services themselves or pay extra to have such services contracted. Although the family members would like to pursue this matter, or move residents to another facility, no other skilled nursing facility options are available in the Smithville area for clients with Medicare as their sole funding source.

Your program has some funding available to provide education to clients and staff of skilled nursing facilities. You are concerned, however, about the fact that previous attempts by your staff to provide this service have been declined by the operators of Sunny Acres.

Questions

1) Discuss additional assessment data needed and how you will go about gathering the data.

2) Present host, agent, and environmental factors, based on data presented in this scenario.
   - Host

   - Agent

   - Environment

3) Discuss interventions that your program may perform at the following levels of prevention:
   - Primary

- Secondary

- Tertiary

4) How will you evaluate the effects of your interventions?

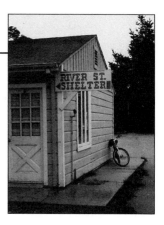

9.13 CASE STUDY

PEDICULOSIS IN HOMELESS SHELTERS

SCENARIO

As a public health nurse working for the Capitol City Health Department you are assigned to
rotate through three shelters for the homeless
once each week. Your role is to assess physical
and metal health issues, health education, basic
first aid, and appropriate referrals. In recent
weeks you have noticed that individuals stay-
ing in a particular homeless shelter have complained of an increased incidence of pediculosis capitis and pubis.

The shelter is operated by an interfaith religious organization. Twelve
religious groups are members of this organization (churches, synagogues,
mosques). Each agency assumes responsibility for operating the shelter
three to four times a month. The hours of operation for the shelter are from
5:00 PM until 10:00 AM. Clients are provided an evening meal, a cot and
blankets, and a morning meal. Hot showers are available in the morning,
with clients rotating through the two showers in the shelter.

Funding and oversight of this program are provided by a volunteer organization working with officials in city government.

Available assessment data related to the problems include:

- Inclement weather has led to an increase in clients requesting shelter.
- Many of these clients would otherwise camp in the wilderness or
  sleep on the streets.

Questions

1) Discuss additional assessment data needed to address the issue of pediculosis in the shelter. How you will go about gathering the data?

2) Based on data presented in this scenario, present host, agent, and environmental factors that may be contributing to the problems.
   - Host

   - Agent

   - Environment

3) Discuss interventions your program will perform at the following levels of prevention:
   - Primary

   - Secondary

   - Tertiary

4) How will you evaluate the effects of your interventions?

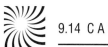 9.14 C A S E S T U D Y

INSURANCE COSTS FOR STRESS AND PREGNANCY LEAVE

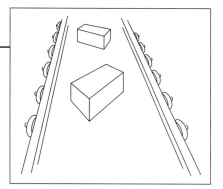

SCENARIO

Metropolis Tool Company is a manufacturing plant that employs 1200 workers. You are an occupational health nurse working for the company.

It has come to your attention that there has been a significant increase in insurance claims for the following conditions:

- Stress-related migraine headaches
- Early pregnancy leave for women experiencing low maternal weight gain

Metropolis Tool Company has been in business for more than 29 years. Recently, competition in the manufacturing industry has increased and the company's executives are looking for ways to cut expenses. Insurance premiums cost the company a considerable amount and rates will increase if the number of claims continues to rise. Your employer recently became aware of the problems leading to increased utilization of disability benefits. He approached you and asked you to "fix" these problems in an expeditious manner.

Available assessment data that may be related to the problems include:

- The plant recently moved to rotating shifts and is now operating around the clock.
- Staff layoffs are predicted within 6 months.
- Increasing corporate competition has led to higher productivity standards.

Questions

1) Discuss additional assessment data needed and how you will go about gathering the data.

2) Present host, agent, and environmental factors, based on data presented in this scenario:
   ● Host

   ● Agent

   ● Environment

3) Discuss interventions your program may perform at the following levels of prevention:
   ● Primary

   ● Secondary

   ● Tertiary

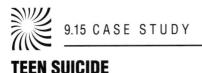 9.15 CASE STUDY

TEEN SUICIDE

SCENARIO

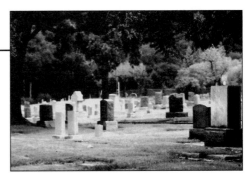

You are a school nurse working at Smithville High School, a rural school with 400 students. In the past year there have been two suicides and two attempted suicides among students in the school.

Assessment data that you feel may be related to this problem include:

- There has been an increase in experimentation with drugs including LSD, marijuana, and alcohol.
- Unemployment levels have risen in the community.
- Most families in the community own personal handguns or rifles.

Questions

1) Discuss additional assessment data needed and how you will go about gathering the data.

2) Present host, agent, and environmental factors, based on data presented in this scenario.
   - Host

   - Agent

   - Environment

3) Discuss interventions your program may perform at the following levels of prevention:
   - Primary

   - Secondary

   - Tertiary

9.16 CASE STUDY

SUPPORT GROUP: LEVELS OF PREVENTION

SCENARIO

You work at the women's health clinic in Jonesville. Your sister recently delivered her third child. When you went to visit her in Metropolis, 2 weeks after the birth, you realized that she was suffering from postpartum depression. Her repeated apologies for the "messy house," her tearfulness and the fact that she reported inability to sleep, all contributed to your conclusion. She told you that she "just felt like dying," that she saw no end in sight. "I can't sleep, I can't clean the house, the kids are acting like brats, and my husband is no help, he just tells me it will all be okay."

Your assistance, along with follow-up by the midwife, enabled your sister to work through her depression. The most significant factor in her recovery, however, has been a support group sponsored by a local women's clinic. You were so impressed with this service that you have decided to begin a support group for individuals affected by postpartum depression.

You would like your employer, the Jonesville Women's Health Clinic, to sponsor the program. When you approach the Board of Directors with your idea, they ask you to come back to them with information supporting your idea.

Questions

1) Discuss potential primary, secondary, and tertiary levels of prevention available in a support group for those affected by postpartum depression.
   - Primary

   - Secondary

   - Tertiary

2) What additional information will assist you in "selling" your idea to the Board?

3) How will you go about gaining input from the community?

References

Feingold, E. (1994). Health care reform—More than cost containment and universal access. *American Journal of Public Health, 84*(5), 727–728.

Sheps, C. G. (1976). Higher education for public health. In *A Report of the Milbank Memorial Fund Commission* (pp. 1–5). New York: Prodist.

CHAPTER 10

Case Management

The Case Manager's Creed

To be a Case Manager

*One must be courteous, diplomatic, caring, shrewd, persua-
sive, assertive, creative, supportive, understanding,
responsible, slow to anger, adaptable, a Sherlock Holmes,
a motivator, up-to-date, good looking, have a good memory, acute business judgment, emotional stability, and the
embodiment of virtue, but with a good working knowledge of sin and evil in all its forms.*

*A Case Manager must understand insurance, electricity,
chemistry, physiology, mechanics, architecture, physics,
bookkeeping, banking, merchandising, selling, trading,
and human nature. A Case Manager must be a coordinator, clinician, coach, therapist, educator, consumer advocate, and administrator.*

*A Case Manager must be a mind reader, a hypnotist and an
athlete, and must know all, see all, and tell nothing and
be everywhere at the same time.*

*They must satisfy the claims managers, the claims examin-
ers, the home office claims department, the underwriting
department, the supervisors, the solicitor, the claimant,
and the state industrial commission.*

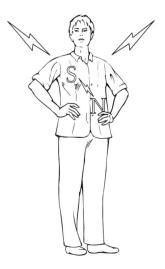

Case management, in its various forms, has been touted as the panacea for the ills of the health care system. To appreciate the role that nurses play in the process of case management, they must have a clear understanding of the definition of the term. Although the definition varies, even among nursing scholars, the universal tenets of case management are presented in this chapter.

REVIEW

"The concept of Case Management is a focus on planned care to integrate, coordinate and advocate for individuals, families, and groups requiring extensive services." (LTU Extension, p. 5)

   I. History of case management (see opposite page)
  II. Authority
 III. Autonomy
 IV. Advocacy
    A. Empowerment
  V. Service coordination
    A. Linkage
    B. Delegation
    C. Supervision
    D. Direct provision of services
 VI. Service monitoring
    A. Quality control
    B. Coordination of health care team
VII. Case management process
    A. Outreach/referral to agency
    B. Assessment

History of Case Management

1863	Case management roots in social work
1900	Case management used in public health practice
1950	Hill Burton Act created community-based regional medical centers
1965	Medicare legislation enacted
	Older Americans Act increased funding for educational programs in gerontology
1970's	Workers compensation case management begun
1975	Diagnosis-related groups (DRGs)
1979	National Committee for Quality Assurance (NCQA) founded by two managed care associations
1990	NCQA became an independent, not-for-profit accrediting agency
1993	Health Security Act (HR 3600) aimed at health care reform
	The goals of the program, as stated by President Clinton, included:
	–Security
	–Simplicity
	–Savings
	–Quality
	–Choice
	–Responsibility
1994	The Medicare Choice Act of 1994 provides Medicare recipients with options for health care coverage

From LTU Extension (pp. 13–15), with permission.

   C. Mutual goal setting
      1. Development of contracts and or care plans
   D. Planning
      1. Identification of available resources
      2. Interagency agreements
   E. Intervention
      1. Service coordination
      2. Service monitoring
      3. Family support and involvement
      4. Outcome evaluation
         a) Quality
         b) Cost

DISCUSSION

Definition

Although nurses may express divergent views about the definition of case management, commonalities exist within the various definitions. The consensus is that a case manager assumes many roles, including that of advocate, facilitator, and fiscal intermediary. The goal of case management is the development and maintenance of a personal relationship with a client in the pursuit of optimal client health. The specific roles of case manager are discussed here.

As an advocate, the case manager works to assist clients in the identification of goals, prioritization of those goals, and identification of resources that will assist in the achievement of desired outcomes. To fully participate in the nurse–client interaction, clients must become empowered. In its most efficacious form, empowerment leads to an integrative power relationship between the nurse and client. Integrative power is defined as "power with another as is evident in an adult relationship" (Bailey, 1990, p. 17). This type of power differs from nutrient power, which is "power for another as a parent has for a child" (Bailey, 1990, p. 17). Only through the acquisition of an integrative power relationship will clients be encouraged to assume responsibility for the direction of their care. This type of nurse–client relationship sets the stage for eventual independent function on the part of the client, who is able to gain access to and use available resources to achieve desired goals.

As a facilitator, the nurse case manager works as a liaison between clients and community resources, agencies (such as hospitals), physicians, and other health care professionals. In addition, the nurse case manager may be in a position to facilitate the enlistment of clients' personal resources, such as family members, neighbors, friends, and individuals from the client's place of worship. The parties must be assessed for their ability and willingness to assist in the care of the client.

As health maintenance organizations (HMOs) become increasingly prevalent, the role of the case manager as the facilitator of health care for clients has expanded. This evolution will ideally lead to more clearly identified roles among health care providers. Additionally, families and friends will be asked to compensate for ancillary services, such as in-home supportive services, which may not be covered under managed care plans. As the facilitators of service provision, nurse case managers must anticipate this trend and prepare to assist those involved in the transition.

Nurses must be skilled in the areas of client and family education to fulfill their role as case manager. Additionally, case managers are asked to educate physicians, insurance companies, and community resource personnel regarding the various financial aspects of the care of clients.

Figure 10-1 depicts the case management funnel, which shows that input is 'filtered' and 'processed' by the nurse case manager who works with clients and colleagues to produce desired outcomes.

In the discussion of "what case management is" one must also consider what case management is not. A case manager is not merely a "gatekeeper," approving or denying client services. Case management is not a solution to every question posed by nurses about their role in health care reform. Neither is case management meant to address and resolve all of the issues affecting clients. Rather, through the tool of case management, clients and nurses work together to identify issues and prioritize those issues both in terms of severity and probability of resolution in the nurse–client relationship.

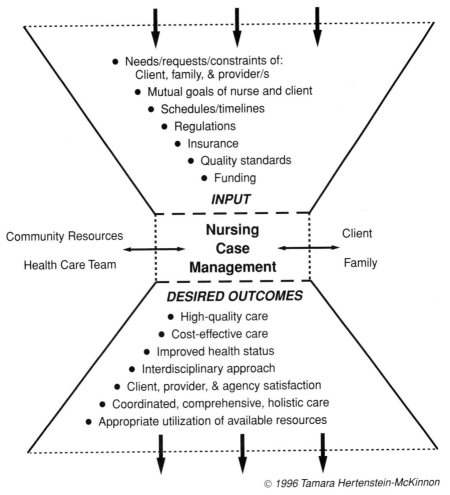

© 1996 Tamara Hertenstein-McKinnon

FIGURE 10-1   The cyclic case management funnel.

Purpose

COST EFFECTIVENESS

Cost effectiveness results from the following aspects of case management:

1. Improved quality of care leading to limitation of disease processes
2. Decreased duplication of services
3. Enlistment of family and other personal support resources
4. Appropriate training of voluntary support persons
5. Identification of available, appropriate low-cost or free resources available to the client
6. Improved adherence to prescribed regime due to client involvement in plan of care

7. Collaborative practice
8. Utilization of advanced practice nurses
9. Improved provider satisfaction resulting from appropriate shared responsibilities leading to decreased provider turnover
10. Focus on prevention
11. Cost shifting (ie, save the insurance company money by using Meals On Wheels rather than more expensive in-home meal preparation service)
12. Education of clients, families, and providers about alternative treatments and low-cost resources
13. Facilitating early discharge from acute facilities
14. Increased knowledge of financial aspects of clients' care, which allows for proactive planning of cost-efficient care

QUALITY IMPROVEMENT

Presented below are ways in which effective case management leads to quality improvement:

1. Effective interdisciplinary communication to enable the health care team to focus on identified desired health outcomes
2. Comprehensive case management beginning before the acute phase of a disease process, allowing sufficient time for identification of mutual goals related to health outcomes and health care team members' contributions
3. Holistic view of clients' issues, problems, and available resources
4. Extensive knowledge of community resources
5. Case conferencing that focuses on outcomes and involves the client and family members

CLIENT SATISFACTION

Clients and their families are encouraged to be active participants in the health care team. Case managers work with clients and families to identify and work toward mutual goals. Case managers gear their approach to each client's unique needs.

STREAMLINING

Decreased fragmentation and duplication occurs through coordination of service provision by all involved parties. Fostering collegial relationships and delineating clear lines of responsibility, including boundaries of expertise, are critical for achievement of this goal.

Although cost saving through the use of case management has been documented, the sense that clients experience improved outcomes is an area that warrants further nursing research.

APPROPRIATE USE OF INTERNAL AND EXTERNAL RESOURCES

To foster independence on the part of the client, the nurse case manager must work with clients and communities to identify available resources. Identification of appropriate, available resources requires a clear understanding of the issues facing clients. Examples of internal resources include personal and family strengths. Examples of external resources include community, societal resources that are available to the client, given her or his particular situation.

Involvement

PROVIDERS

Case management services have been provided for many years by professionals such as nurses and social workers. Lay case managers function in a variety of settings such as public health programs and community clinics. The lack of mandatory certification, along with ambiguity about the definition of case management, have resulted in role confusion, particularly with the recent focus on case management in the area of managed care. "The American Nurses Association recommends the baccalaureate degree with several years of clinical experience as the minimum requirement for nurse case managers" (American Nurses Association [ANA] Task Force on Case Management, 1988).

Contrary to the impression given by the quote at the beginning of this chapter, a nurse case manager must possess specific skills and meet certain requirements. Examples include:

- Licensure as a registered nurse
- Bachelor's or master's degree requirement for some agencies
- Ability to practice autonomously
- Flexibility and creativity
- Strong communication skills for
  - Interdisciplinary team coordination
    Working as a liaison among clients, families, providers, and funding sources
  - Possible required certification as a case manager (refer to Appendix B)
  - Clinical expertise (ie, nursing specialty such as pediatrics, rehabilitation, or utilization review and quality assurance)

CLIENTS

Examples of client groups appropriate for case management services include:

- High volume/population focused
  - Maternal-child health
    Prenatal
    Elderly

- High-risk groups
  - High-risk infants
- Inpatient
  - Discharge planning
  - Utilization review
- Disease specific
  - Chronic or long-term illnesses
- Occupational health
- High cost
  - Improper utilization of services (ie, frequent emergency room visits)
  - Technology dependent
  - Acquired immunodeficiency syndrome (AIDS)
  - Transplants
- High acuity
- Life-threatening, terminal disease, newly diagnosed

As a rule, one case manager should be designated as the lead, or primary, case manager. Along with this title comes the responsibility of coordinating all other individuals and entities providing services to the identified clients. Most often the primary case manager is an employee or representative of an insurance company. Although this practice has been questioned, the funding source's representative is often best suited to coordinate health care services because many decisions about provision of care will be incumbent on funding.

Principles

Although the principles of case management have been used by nurses, social workers, and other professional for many years, the term case management has become a buzz word accompanying health care reform and managed care. Case management does indeed present nursing with new and exciting opportunities to demonstrate its capacity for autonomous practice. Case management, however, is not a panacea for the nursing profession and many unresolved issues remain. The most important of these include ambiguous or conflicting definitions and a lack of standards for educational preparation of nurse case managers.

To truly benefit from the opportunities afforded the profession, nurses must form a common definition of nursing case management. Similarly, the educational preparation standards for nurse case managers must be defined by nurses, or these requirements will be defined for them by other power structures such as physicians, hospitals, insurance companies, or governmental agencies. Including case management principles and practicums in the curricula of nursing education will assist the profession in achieving these goals. If nurses are not proactive now, they will be forced to be reactive in the future, when the opportunity to influence the course of professional nursing case management may be limited.

USE OF THE NURSING PROCESS

I. Assessment
   A. Evaluate proposed/prescribed care
   B. Analyze options
   C. Analyze cost of various approaches
   D. Determine client/family goals for care
      1. Short-term goals
      2. Long-term goals
   E. Assess coverage from payment source
   F. Gather input
      1. Providers
      2. Resources
II. Statement of issues
   A. Problems and strengths
      1. Mutually identified
III. Plan
   A. Appropriate use of interdisciplinary team members
   B. Direct care to meet desired outcome criteria
   C. Cost-effective approach
      1. Cost savings
      2. Cost shifting
IV. Implementation
   A. Case conferencing
   B. Service coordination/service provision
   C. Appropriate use of services
V. Evaluation
   A. Based on outcome criteria/satisfaction of
      1. Client
      2. Family
      3. Providers
      4. Funding sources
   B. Quality of care
   C. Cost containment
VI. Case conferencing
VII. Cost analysis

A *case conference* provides an opportunity for all those involved in a client's care to discuss their role in the provision of coordinated, holistic client care. Ideally, both internal and external resources will be represented during the case conference. During the case conference, the identified primary case manager assumes responsibility for the direction of client care. This is based on factors such as client's desired outcome and available resources.

Formula 10-1 (used in 10.2 to 10.5 Case Studies) is a case conference worksheet used to assist in the coordination of the case conferencing process.

Cost analysis is an important component of case management. In an effort to provide high-quality, cost-effective care, case managers are often asked to provide alternatives to prescribed plans of care. The cost analysis worksheet presented here will allow students to develop alternative treatment plans and to analyze those plans in terms of cost and projected outcomes.

Formula 10-2 (used in 10.6 to 10.8 Case Studies) is a worksheet used to assist in the analysis of costs of treatment plans.

Case Studies and Exercises

Responses to the following case studies and exercises reflect the ability to:

1. Plan and coordinate an interdisciplinary case conference.
2. Identify components of the case management funnel, including input, case management activities, and desired outcomes.
3. Analyze case costs.
4. Outline an alternative treatment plan to reduce the cost of client care.

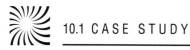 10.1 CASE STUDY

MEDICAL-SURGICAL: DIABETES AND DECUBITI

SCENARIO

You are a nurse case manager working for the County Managed Care System in Brownsville. Your duties include service coordination, service monitoring, and cost containment. You have a caseload ranging from 200 to 250 individuals. You rarely do home visits; most of your work is done via telephone conversations.

The majority of your work involves the review of medical bills and requests for service. You are responsible for determination of medical eligibility for payment of bills for the managed care clients in your caseload.

Assessment Data

In reviewing your records you note that within the past 8 months you have authorized 10 inpatient stays for one of your clients, Mrs. Johansen. Mrs. Johansen was discharged last week after a 4-day inpatient hospitalization.

Mrs. Johansen is a 67 year-old woman with poorly managed diabetes mellitus and a history of stage II pressure sores. The purpose of her inpatient stays have been to get the diabetes under control and to treat pressure sores.

Mrs. Johansen is divorced and lives alone in downtown Brownsville. She had been active in her church and is concerned that her volunteer work has suffered due to her medical condition. Mrs. Johansen has two sons living in Capitol City.

Problem Statement

- Diabetes mellitus with poor control
- Impaired tissue integrity (recurrent pressure sores)
- High cost of treatment resulting from repeated inpatient hospitalizations
- Potential for social isolation
- Potential for noncompliance with therapeutic regimen related to the complexity and chronic nature of diabetes

Plan

SERVICE COORDINATION AND MONITORING

Coordinate efforts of all currently involved and potentially beneficial resources (personal and community). Identify responsible parties for various aspects of care for Mrs. Johansen.

As a service coordinator your role is to identify specific needs of Mrs. Johansen and to ensure that service providers and appropriate community resource agencies are working with the client toward mutually identified goals. The specific course of treatment for each service is determined by the service provider and your client. This approach will decrease fragmentation and duplication in the provision of care for Mrs. Johansen.

Implementation

Action	Rationale
Examine alternatives to inpatient hospitalization (ie, provision of home health nursing)	Cost containment
	Client comfort
	Long-term improvement in outcome with holistic approach
	Assessment of ways in which client's lifestyle and home environment may contribute to medical problems will lead to patient teaching, which will specifically address those issues.
Coordinate with physician	Home care must be deemed appropriate by physician and prescribed as a treatment measure
Obtain information from hospital nurses and discharge planner	Gather assessment data related to patient's situation (ie, family support)
	Evaluate data regarding self-care and knowledge of disease processes

(continued)

Action	Rationale
Involve client in planning and decision-making process.	Assess desire for home care for the purposes of assessment, monitoring, and patient teaching (this step comes after ensuring that home care is a viable option for the client). Is there a preferred home health agency of those covered on the managed care plan? What are her goals related to these diagnoses?
Set mutual goals with client (ie, decrease hospitalizations and incidence of pressure sores by keeping diabetes under control (blood sugars consistently between 130–150 mg/dL). Identify possible resources which may assist in attainment of goal (resources which Mrs. Johansen feels comfortable with).	
Coordinate with home health agency discuss plans for attainment of mutual goals.	
Identify and coordinate with appropriate community resources (as requested by Mrs. Johansen): • Meals On Wheels • In-home supportive services • Church members • Family members	No identified primary caregiver May supply diabetic diet at minimal charge Provide assistance in maintenance of home by helping with chores, etc Psychological support Psychological support

Evaluation

CLIENT OUTCOMES

GOAL

After 8 months of home health nursing intervention along with ancillary supportive services:

1. Mrs. Johansen will express satisfaction with approach to care.
2. Blood sugar readings will indicate control of diabetes (blood sugar levels of 130–150 mg/dL).
3. Early indications of pressure sores will be identified and treated leading to the prevention of further pressure sores.
4. Inpatient hospitalization will not be needed.

5. Ongoing communication with parties involved with Mrs. Johansen's care will ensure identification of new actual or potential problems.

FISCAL OUTCOMES

Plan A: Inpatient Option

Service		Cost (estimate)
Hospitalization over 8 months (10 admissions, 4 days/admission, $200 per day)	**Total Cost**	$8,000

Plan B: In-Home Management Option

Service		Cost (estimate)
Home Health • Week 1 1 week 4 visits 2 h each = 8 h • Week 2 1 week 3 visits 2 h each = 6 h • Week 3–6 4 weeks 2 visits 2 h each = 16 h Managed care rate for nursing care in home: $35/h		$1,050
Meals On Wheels $2 per day × 8 months (34 weeks)		$476
In-home Support Services 16 h per week × $6.00 per h × 8 months (34 weeks)		$3,264
Cost of this option (in-home)(for 8 months)	**Total Cost**	$4,790

COST COMPARISON

- 8 months with inpatient hospitalizations: $8,000
- 8 months with in-home management: $4,790
- Potential cost savings/cost shifting: $3,210

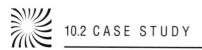 10.2 C A S E S T U D Y

INTERDISCIPLINARY CASE CONFERENCING

Questions

Consider 10.1 Case Study.

1) As the primary case manager, who will you involve in the Mrs. Johansen's case conferences? Provide rationale for your responses.

2) What are your goals for the initial case conference? What issues do you plan to address?

3) What additional information must you obtain about Mrs. Johansen, in the following categories, to provide appropriate case management in the home environment? Discuss your approach to gathering information related to these categories:
   - Diagnosis

   - Client

   - Family

   - Aggregate

- Community

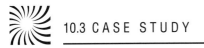 10.3 CASE STUDY

PEDIATRIC CEREBRAL PALSY

SCENARIO

You are a case manager with Capitol City Hospital's discharge planning unit. Today's case conference focuses on Marietta, a 4-year-old child with severe cerebral palsy. Marietta lives with her parents and her 7-year-old sister in an apartment complex in downtown Capitol City.

Identified problems include:

- Failure to thrive
- Developmental delay
- Legally blind
- Poor-fitting wheelchair
- Contractures
- Mother experiencing difficulty with nasogastric tube feedings
- Parents undergoing divorce
- Sibling with attention deficit disorder (ADD)
- Family has no means of reliable transportation
- Mother quit her job (4 years ago) to provide total care to Marietta; the family income had been supplemented by a pension plan buyout; that money is nearly gone.

Marietta was admitted to the hospital for treatment of excoriation of the buttocks and evaluation of parenteral nutrition needs. Marietta and her family receive support and direct services from several community agencies including:

- Easter Seals
- Capitol City Regional Center (supportive services for developmentally delayed client and their families)
- Health Department
    - District nurse home visits
- County Mental Health Services
    - Counseling for parents
- Physician's prescription
    - Trial period of total parenteral nutrition in the home
    - Placement in foster care or pediatric skilled nursing facility due to long-standing failure to thrive

- Funding
  - Payer, County Managed Care, does not pay for home health services

Questions

Use Formula 10-1 as a guide in addressing this case.

FORMULA 10-1

Case Conference Worksheet

TEAM MEMBERS

- Primary case manager: _____
- Team members:

  _____

  _____

  _____

  _____

ASSESSMENT

Client information (assessment data provided by team members)
- Medical:

- Psychological:
    Strengths

    Problems

- Payor/s:

STATEMENT OF ISSUES

- State problems (in order of priority):

- List strengths/assets:

(continued)

FORMULA 10-1 (Continued)

PLAN

Action	Responsible Party/Agency	Due Date

IMPLEMENTATION

Each team member capitalizes on resources and areas of expertise to act upon plan.

EVALUATION

Were desired outcomes achieved?
- Why?

- Why not?

> Return as a team and evaluate and strategize about necessary alterations to plan. Determine what additional information will assist in revision of plan.

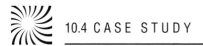 10.4 CASE STUDY

MEDICAL-SURGICAL: BURNS

SCENARIO

You are an occupational health nurse consultant working for a large construction firm in Metropolis. Steve is a 42-year-old construction worker who is an employee of the company. Steve suffered extensive second- and third-degree burns in an industrial accident 2 months ago. He has been in the burn and rehabilitation units of Metropolis Hospital until last week.

Steve's issues are:

1. He has moderate contractures of both hands.
2. His wife is at home with the couple's 6-month-old daughter.
3. Steve wants to return to work as soon as possible.
4. His physician and physical therapist have both advised against manual labor for at least one full year.
5. Steve's immune system remains compromised as a result of the accident.

Goals of Case Management

1. Assessment and maintenance of integrity of each body system
2. Prevention of infection
3. Education
    Asepsis
    Signs and symptoms of infection
4. Nutritional management and maintenance
    Fluid and electrolyte balance
5. Pain management
6. Maximize physical mobility
7. Identify self-care needs
8. Psychological assessment and support
    Appropriate referrals to assist client/family in dealing with
        grief, social isolation, anxiety, and fears
    Alterations in family processes

Questions

Coordinate the case conference, using Formula 10-1, based on the information provided in this scenario.

FORMULA 10-1

Case Conference Worksheet

TEAM MEMBERS

- Primary case manager: _____
- Team members:

    _____

    _____

    _____

    _____

(continued)

FORMULA 10-1 (Continued)

ASSESSMENT

Client information (assessment data provided by team members)
- Medical:

- Psychological:
    Strengths

    Problems

- Payor/s:

STATEMENT OF ISSUES

- State problems (in order of priority):

- List strengths/assets:

PLAN

Action	Responsible Party/Agency	Due Date

IMPLEMENTATION

Each team member capitalizes on resources and areas of expertise to act upon plan.

(continued)

FORMULA 10-1 (Continued)

EVALUATION

Were desired outcomes achieved?
- Why?

- Why not?

      Return as a team and evaluate and strategize about necessary alterations to plan. Determine what additional information will assist in revision of plan.

 10.5 CASE STUDY

AIDS SEROPOSITIVE CLIENT
AND SERONEGATIVE CAREGIVER

SCENARIO

You are a case manager working with a home health agency in Capitol City. Your client is JB, a 33-year-old man who has been positive for human immunodeficiency virus (HIV) for 4 years. JB was recently diagnosed with AIDS.

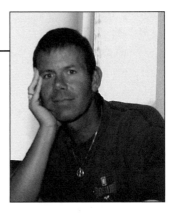

JB lives at home with Doug, his partner of 6 years. Doug has received serial HIV antibody testing and remains HIV antibody negative.

    The issues facing JB at this time include:

1. Recent diagnosis of AIDS
2. *Pneumocystis carinii* pneumonia
3. Fear of losing his job as a stockbroker due to the illness
4. Immune suppression
5. Limited family support (family lives out of state but is emotionally supportive)
6. Financial constraints (the couple recently purchased a home, which used most of their savings)
7. Fear of death and dying

Questions

Using the case conference format in Formula 10-1, coordinate this case.

FORMULA 10-1

Case Conference Worksheet

TEAM MEMBERS

- Primary case manager: _____
- Team members:

_____

_____

_____

_____

ASSESSMENT

Client information (assessment data provided by team members)
- Medical:

- Psychological:
    Strengths

    Problems

- Payor/s:

STATEMENT OF ISSUES

- State problems (in order of priority):

- List strengths/assets:

PLAN

Action	Responsible Party/Agency	Due Date

(continued)

FORMULA 10-1 (Continued)

PLAN

Action	Responsible Party/Agency	Due Date

IMPLEMENTATION

Each team member capitalizes on resources and areas of expertise to act upon plan.

EVALUATION

Were desired outcomes achieved?
• Why?

• Why not?

Return as a team and evaluate and strategize about necessary alterations to plan.
Determine what additional information will assist in revision of plan.

 10.6 CASE STUDY

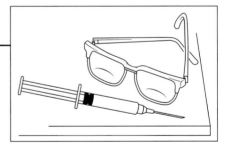

GERONTOLOGY/MEDICAL-SURGICAL: DIABETES AND MACULAR DEGENERATION

SCENARIO

Mrs. Hargrove is a 78-year-old woman with type II diabetes mellitus and macular degeneration. She has had several hospitalizations over the past few months and has been treated for loss of integrity of the epidermis. Mrs. Hargrove has suffered hematomas and lacerations in the process of performing activities of daily living (ADLs) in her home. Her impaired vision, along with diabetes, have combined to make her susceptible to injuries and concurrent integumentary problems.

Mrs. Hargrove is a widow who, until recently, resided in Metropolis with her daughter Mary, aged 56, and Mary's husband, Ted, aged 58. The couple has five children, ranging in age from 18 to 32 years. One month ago Mary's employer transferred her to a new position overseas in Germany. Although they were reluctant to leave Mrs. Hargrove, they felt that the grandchildren, three of whom remained in Metropolis, could assist with Mrs. Hargrove's needs. The grandchildren living in Metropolis are:

- Jared, age 32, lives with his partner, Tom. They both work at a large supermarket in Metropolis.
- Tracy, 19, is single and a law school student in Metropolis.
- Tony, 21, attends a local junior college and works part-time as a mechanic. Tony lives with his grandmother, Mrs. Hargrove, and assists her with shopping and home maintenance. Tony has been spending less time at home recently because he has increased his coursework at the junior college.

Mrs. Hargrove is adamant that she will remain in her home. She reportedly told her physician "I'd rather die than leave." Mrs. Hargrove's current admission follows a fall down three stairs from her front porch. She told the nurse in the emergency room, at the time of her admission, that as she bent over to get the morning paper, she misjudged the distance and tumbled down the steps. Mrs. Hargrove suffered a small laceration to her right knee and one to her right shoulder. At the time of admission it was also noted that Mrs. Hargrove had problems related to foot and toenail care and hygiene.

Her physician has proposed the following course of treatment:

- Four days inpatient
  - To monitor and educate client about blood sugar levels
  - To treat lacerations and assess for signs of infection
- Four home health visits
  - To assess and educate about safety hazards in the home
  - To identify resources to assist in ADLs

Her insurance coverage includes:

- Medicaid
- Medicare
- Pension plan from her late-husband's employer ($120/month)

Your role: Medicare Case Manager

Questions

Refer to Figure 10-1, case management funnel.

1) Identify the input that you, as a case manager, will address in this scenario.

2) Discuss appropriate case management given this scenario.

3) Given the information available to you, what do you consider to be desired outcomes in this scenario?

Analyze this case using Formula 10-2.
Your role: Medicare Case Manager

FORMULA 10-2

Case Cost Analysis Worksheet

I. PLAN A
PROPOSED/PRESCRIBED COURSE OF TREATMENT
(Length of inpatient stay, etc.)

Service	*Cost (estimate*)*
Total Cost:	**$**

(continued)

FORMULA 10-2 (Continued)

II: PLAN B
ALTERNATIVE COURSE OF TREATMENT WITH CASE MANAGEMENT

Service	Cost (estimate*)
Total Cost:	$

Analysis of Alternatives

Desired Outcome

Plan A	Plan B

Cost (estimate)*

Plan A: $	Plan B: $

(continued)

FORMULA 10-2 (Continued)

DISCUSSION:

Estimate cost based on prevailing rates in your community.

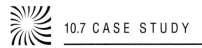 10.7 CASE STUDY

MEDICAL-SURGICAL: COLOSTOMY

SCENARIO

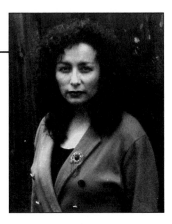

Maria is a 28-year-old Hispanic woman who speaks only Spanish. Maria lives with her husband and their 12-year-old son in Smithville. She has a large extended family living in Brownsville. After many years of problems related to ulcerative colitis, Maria's physicians have determined that she is in need of a colostomy. Maria will be admitted 1 week from today for the procedure. Her physician's recommended course of treatment is:

   Day 1: Preadmit for laboratory and x-ray evaluations
   Day 2: Surgery and postoperative
   Days 3–5: Recovery. Monitoring and postoperative teaching (hygiene, care of ostomy, nutrition education and self-care)

Maria and her husband work together delivering newspapers in Smithville. They have a large territory and generally adhere to the following schedule:

- Fold and sort papers from 3:00 AM until 5:00 AM
- Drive their route from 5:30 AM until 8:00 AM
- Drive their son to school
- Rest
- Pick up their son from school at 2:30 PM
- Work together delivering the Brownsville evening paper to a smaller, rural route from 3:00 PM until 6:00 PM

Although Maria and her family have faced her previous health problems as a united front, there is a great deal of concern and embarrassment related to the prospect of living with a colostomy. The couple's son, Jaime, serves as the family's interpreter. Through Jaime, Maria informed her physician that she would like to have postponed the surgery if possible, that she did not feel the family was ready. After a lengthy discussion with her physician in which he impressed on her the gravity of her situation, however, Maria agreed to proceed with the surgery as scheduled.

Your role: Utilization Review Nurse for Managed Care Operation.

Questions

Refer to Figure 10-1, case management funnel.

1) Identify the input that you, as a case manager, will address in this scenario.

2) Discuss appropriate case management given this scenario.

3) Given the information available to you, what do you consider to be desired outcomes in this scenario?

Analyze this case using Formula 10-2.
Your role: Utilization Review Nurse for Managed Care Operation

FORMULA 10-2

Case Cost Analysis Worksheet

I. PLAN A
PROPOSED/PRESCRIBED COURSE OF TREATMENT
(Length of inpatient stay, etc.)

Service	*Cost (estimate*)*

(continued)

FORMULA 10-2 (Continued)

Service	Cost (estimate*)
Total Cost:	$

II: PLAN B
ALTERNATIVE COURSE OF TREATMENT WITH CASE MANAGEMENT

Service	Cost (estimate*)
Total Cost:	$

(continued)

FORMULA 10-2 (Continued)

Analysis of Alternatives

Desired Outcome

Plan A	Plan B

Cost (estimate*)

Plan A: $	Plan B: $

DISCUSSION:

*Estimate cost based on prevailing rates in your community.

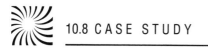

10.8 CASE STUDY

MENTAL HEALTH: STRESS

SCENARIO

Amy works as a child care provider at the corporate office of a large multi-national bank in downtown Metropolis. You work as an occupational health nurse for the bank. The child care center in which Amy works has

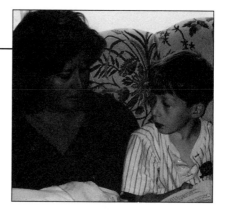

38 children, ranging in age from 2 months to 6 years. Amy and her col-

leagues are paid $7.00/h plus benefits (approximately $2.50/h). Amy's duties include:

- Opening the center at 6:00 AM
- Signing children in
- Checking individual children's special needs for the day (ie, medications)
- Staffing the newborn section (children aged 2–6 months) from 9:00 AM until 12 noon (3–5 children);
- Break from 10:30 to 11:30
- Assisting other staff members in feeding all children 12:00 noon until 2:00 PM
- Assist with naps from 2:00 PM until 3:00 PM

In recent months Amy has expressed concerns about an increased level of stress related to her job. When the problem was presented to you, you facilitated Amy's access to the counseling services offered by your company's employee assistance program (EAP). Despite intervention by counselors working with the EAP, Amy felt that her job-related stress had continued to escalate. Amy was then seen by a psychiatrist who placed her on disability for 6 weeks due to job-related stress.

Six weeks have now passed. Amy has undergone intensive psychiatric counseling. Although the psychiatrist feels that Amy's stress level has decreased somewhat and that she has developed additional coping skills, he feels that her condition warrants an additional 6-week disability leave.

Your goal is to develop a plan that will allow Amy to return to work as soon as possible. You will work with Amy, the employer, and the psychiatrist to modify Amy's workload or restructure her job to accommodate her disability.

Questions

Refer to Figure 10-1, case management funnel.

1) Identify the input which you, as a case manager, will address in this scenario.

2) Discuss appropriate case management given this scenario.

3) Given the information available to you, what do you consider to be desired outcomes in this scenario?

Analyze this case using Formula 10-2.
Your role: Occupational Health Nurse

FORMULA 10-2

Case Cost Analysis Worksheet

I. PLAN A
PROPOSED/PRESCRIBED COURSE OF TREATMENT
(Length of inpatient stay, etc.)

Service	Cost (estimate*)
Total Cost:	$

(continued)

FORMULA 10-2 (Continued)

II: PLAN B
ALTERNATIVE COURSE OF TREATMENT WITH CASE MANAGEMENT

Service	*Cost (estimate*)*
Total Cost:	**$**

Analysis of Alternatives

Desired Outcome

Plan A	Plan B

Cost (estimate*)

Plan A: $	Plan B: $

(continued)

FORMULA 10-2 (Continued)

DISCUSSION:

Estimate cost based on prevailing rates in your community.

References

American Nurses Association Task Force on Case Management in Nursing. (1988). *Nursing Case Management* (Publication No. NS-32). Kansas City, MO: Author.

Bailey, B. (1990). The concepts of empowerment and care of the hospice patient and family. *Journal of Home Health Nursing Practice, 3*(1), 16–22.

Learning Tree University (LTU Extension). (1996). *Introduction to Case Management.* Chatsworth, CA: Author.

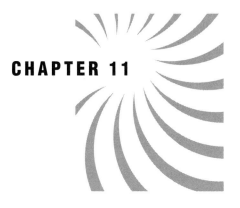

CHAPTER 11

Ethical Issues in Community Health Nursing

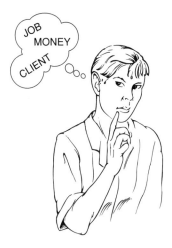

The Florence Nightingale Pledge

I solemnly pledge myself before God and in presence of this assembly;

To pass my life in purity and to practice my profession faith-fully.

I will abstain from whatever is deleterious and mischievous and will not take or knowingly administer any harmful drug.

I will do all in my power to maintain and elevate the stan-dard of my profession and will hold in confidence all per-

sonal matters committed to my keeping and family affairs coming to my knowledge in the practice of my calling.

With loyalty will I endeavor to aid the physician in his work, and devote myself to the welfare of those committed to my care.

(Bishop, from Davis & Aroskar, 1978, pp. 12–13)

As fiscal constraints exert increasing influence over nursing practice, unique ethical dilemmas are presented. Nurses face situations in which they have allegiance to numerous entities, including their employer, the payer of services; clients; families; and personal and professional morals. Chapter 11 addresses the issues of advocacy, autonomy, and accountability as they relate to ethical community health nursing practice.

REVIEW _____

  I. Ethics
   A. Definition: "The rules or standards of conduct governing the members of a profession" (*Webster's II*, 1984, p. 445)
   B. Nursing ethics
      1. Nurse practice acts
      2. Fundamental responsibilities of the nurse
         a) Promotion of health
         b) Prevention of illness
         c) Restoration of health
         d) Alleviation of suffering (Davis & Aroskar, 1978, p. 13)
   C. Personal ethics
      1. Nurse
      2. Client
   D. Societal ethics
      1. Employing agency
         a) Managed care
      2. Governmental
         a) Funding
 II. Advocacy
III. Autonomy
 IV. Accountability
   A. Obligation
      1. Primary responsibility of the community health nurse
      2. Legal, moral, and ethical obligations of the profession
      3. Reporting
      4. Informed consent

V. Potential sources of ethical conflicts in community health nursing
   A. Values and principles
      1. Client
      2. Individual nurse
      3. Nursing organization
      4. Agency
      5. Society
VI. Terms and theories related to nursing ethics
   A. Veracity
   B. Justice
   C. Beneficence
   D. Confidentiality
   E. Ethical theories (Davis & Aroskar, 1978, p. 28)
      1. Egoism
      2. Deontology or formalism
      3. Utilitarianism
      4. Obligation (Frankena)
      5. Ideal observer (Firth)
      6. Justice as fairness (Rawls)

DISCUSSION

Ethical considerations related to issues such as client advocacy and cost containment are not unique to community health nursing. Nurses have long struggled with moral and ethical decisions related to the provision of quality client care. The introduction of health care reform measures, however, has presented new and unique challenges to the field of community health nursing. Nurses' allegiance to the profession, the employer, the client, and themselves are increasingly called into question.

Where does the primary responsibility of the nurse lie? What is the universal code of nursing ethics? Who can nurses turn to with difficult ethical decisions? These and other questions have plagued the field of nursing since the days when Florence Nightingale penned her pledge. The difficulty in responding to these questions lies in the fact that ethical tenets are often in conflict and that there is seldom one clearly "good" or "right" solution. This chapter presents a brief overview of nursing ethics. The case studies that follow will assist the learner in evaluation of personal ethics. This is also an opportunity for the learner to identify resources, which will assist the learner in responding to ethical questions. These activities will prepare the learner for the inevitable ethical conflicts that will ensue in the practice of community health nursing.

Advocacy

To be an advocate is "to plead in another's behalf" (*Webster's II*, 1984, p. 81). Advocacy in community health nursing presents continual challenges, both in terms of its definition and application. If advocacy in its literal sense means doing for or fighting for someone, how are clients encouraged to move toward independence and self-determination? In the acute care setting nurses may be asked to act in the best interest of clients who are unable to act on their own behalf. In the community setting, however, most clients are in a position of thinking and acting for themselves. In this situation, the nurse who "does for" the client and family something that they are capable of doing for themselves may actually be performing a disservice to the client. Rather than acting for families, therefore, it is often in the best interest of clients to assist them in the performance of the task and to work with them to develop the ability to perform the tasks and advocate for themselves.

In a more general sense, advocacy for clients in the community health environment involves working together to meet the needs of aggregates and populations. At this level of advocacy the nurse works with systems such as political systems, or within the employing agency, to address the needs of the population being served. In this role the nurse may teach community classes, address the county Board of Supervisors, or meet with agency representatives or other influential groups serving their population. Working to advocate for necessary change requires nurses to be keenly aware of the political environment. Most importantly, nurses must be in touch with their clients' needs to advocate for changes that will be in the best interest of those involved.

Autonomy

Autonomy is "the quality or condition of being self-governing" (*Webster's II*, 1984, p. 140). As with advocacy, autonomy has unique implications in the field of community health nursing. Following are examples of the rights held by the various entities involved in the relationships of community health:

- Client
  - Privacy
  - Respect
  - Self-determination
  - Personal responsibility
  - Informed consent
  - Right to receive or refuse treatment
      Advanced directives
      Alternative treatments
  - "Bill of Rights"
- Nurse
  - Personal and professional decision-making affecting:
      Provision of quality client care
      Work environment
  - Accountability
- Society
  - Cost-effective health care

Community health nurses are particularly challenged to respect their clients' individuality and uniqueness because they practice on the client's 'turf'. Nurses strive toward the identification and achievement of mutual goals by allowing for, and encouraging, self-determination. Conflicts arise when self-determination is subordinated by safety concerns for the client or the general public. In such instances nurses may be called on to enforce legal measures (ie, quarantine) or may be in a position to work with clients to change behaviors.

Accountability

Nurses are *accountable* for actions that they "ought" to take in the best interest of clients. Nurses are *responsible* for actions that they are required to take in the interest of clients. Nurses' legal responsibilities include, but are not limited to, mandated reporting such as in the cases of child abuse or neglect. The distinction between accountability and responsibility is often critical in matters of ethical debate. Although a nurse may feel a sense of duty to intervene in a particular manner, it may not be required. Conversely, although a nurse may fear that dissemination of client information may lead to mistrust or anger on the part of the client, the nurse may be obligated to divulge such information. Clarifying responsibilities and obligations will assist the nurse in sorting out complex issues in which obligations are at odds with one another (ie, responsibility to client versus responsibility to society).

Determination of the nurse's primary obligation is often a difficult matter. In any given community health scenario, the nurse may be accountable to any of the following entities:

1. Self
2. Nursing profession
3. Individual client
4. Family
5. Aggregate
6. Population
7. Agency
8. Society
9. Funding source

Potential resources for ethical dilemmas in community health nursing practice include:

- Self-awareness, which will assist the nurse in identification of personal beliefs and values that may be influencing a situation
- Personal resources such as clergy and mentors for resolution of issues of a purely personal nature
- Professional standards to guide the nurse in identifying accountability and responsibilities in cases with ethical conflict
- Agencies offering expert advice in terms of ethicists, counselors, or mentors

Case Studies and Exercises

Responses to case studies and exercises reflect the ability to:

1. Acknowledge and identify actual and potential ethical dilemmas.
2. Analyze complex scenarios and discuss the nurse's primary responsibility.
3. Explain accountability of nurses in various roles as it relates to specific scenarios.
4. Provide examples of nurses' roles in advocating for clients.
5. Define empowerment.
6. Analyze the pros and cons of autonomous nursing practice.
7. Consider personal reactions to ethical dilemmas.
8. Identify resources available to assist nurses in the consideration of ethical issues.
9. Debate ethical issues related to health care.

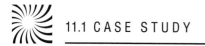 11.1 CASE STUDY

PEDIATRICS: CONGENITAL CARDIAC DEFECTS

SCENARIO

Jacklyn is a 4-year-old girl with congenital cardiac defects. Jacklyn's father is Native American and her mother is Chinese American. Jacklyn lives with her mother and three older stepbrothers (from her mother's first marriage) in a low-income apartment complex in Metropolis. Jacklyn's father is incarcerated for armed robbery and is scheduled to be released from prison in a month. The family has no relatives in this state. The closest relative is Jacklyn's maternal grandmother who lives in a small farming community more than 2000 miles away.

Since birth, Jacklyn has undergone seven cardiac surgeries. The family receives the following services:

- Aid to Families with Dependent Children
- Medicaid
- Social Security (for Jacklyn)
- Food stamps
- Low-income housing

In recent months Jacklyn's mother, Anna, has had increasing difficulty dealing with the stress of limited income, Jacklyn's illness, single parenthood, and personal recovery from substance abuse (cocaine addiction). Recently Anna was arrested for prostitution. At the time of her arrest, police found a large amount of crack cocaine in Anna's possession.

Currently, the family's circumstances are as follows:

1. Anna was sentenced to 2 years in prison and is to begin serving her sentence in 1 week.
2. Jacklyn's stepbrothers will stay with their father and his new wife in Smithville.
3. Jacklyn is scheduled for surgery in 3 weeks; she has weekly visits at Metropolis Hospital before surgery.
4. Jacklyn's case has been under evaluation by Medicaid managed care due to long-term major expenditure. The necessity for some of the surgeries has been questioned by the managed care operation's new administrator. He has challenged Jacklyn's physician to demonstrate that this procedure is more than simply a palliative measure, that it will have some long-term beneficial outcome.
5. Anna's mother, who suffers from angina and arthritis, has offered to care for Jacklyn.
6. Jacklyn's father is requesting an early release from prison to care for the child.
7. Anna's request for release from jail time, due to extenuating circumstances, has been denied.

Questions

Placing yourself in the following community health nurse roles, respond to the questions presented.

COMMUNITY HEALTH NURSE ROLES
1) Nurse with the county's foster care program
   - Who is/are your clients?

   - To whom are you accountable and what are your responsibilities?

2) Utilization review nurse for the county's Medicaid managed care program
   - Who is/are your clients?

   - To whom are you accountable and what are your responsibilities?

3) Home health nurse performing Jacklyn's weekly physical assessments in the home
   - Who is/are your clients?

   - To whom are you accountable and what are your responsibilities?

4) District public health nurse
   - Who is/are your clients?

   - To whom are you accountable and what are your responsibilities?

5) Supervising nurse working in the prison housing Jacklyn's father
   - Who is/are your clients?

   - To whom are you accountable and what are your responsibilities?

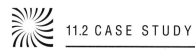 11.2 CASE STUDY

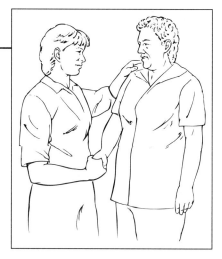

PEDIATRICS: SETTING LIMITS AND IDENTIFYING LINES OF RESPONSIBILITY

SCENARIO

You have recently been hired as the nurse for Smithville Elementary School. You are replacing Nurse Gallinite, who has held the position for the past 35 years. Nurse Gallinite is beloved by students, their families, and the faculty. She has won many awards for her willingness to "go the extra mile" for students. The school administrator, who is your supervisor, has expressed her desire for "things to go on as if Nurse Gallinite had never left us." She has encouraged you "not to rock the boat."

Before leaving her position, Nurse Gallinite informed you that she wanted to fill you in on some of her "special" families. She advised you that these families are unable to manage things on their own, that they will need extra assistance and attention from you to "keep their lives in order." She adds that these families, for various reasons, have "too much going on in their lives," that the children (students at your school) would be the ones to suffer if things were not "taken care of" by you in your role as school nurse.

She gives the example of the Sparks family. The Sparks family consists of:

- Patti, the mother, who is employed as a bank teller in Brownsville
- Jack, the father, who works in an oil refinery outside of Smithville
- Sandra, the 12-year-old daughter, who attends junior high school
- Jack Jr, the 7-year-old son, who attends second grade at Smithville Elementary School

Both Sandra and Jack have been diagnosed with attention deficit disorder. Additionally, Jack has recently been diagnosed as having significant hearing loss in his left ear. These diagnoses have required frequent visits to specialists in Brownsville.

Nurse Gallinite has informed you that these parents were students in Smithville Elementary School years ago and that she is very familiar with their backgrounds. She advises you that they "worked very hard to get where they are today." She adds that she has helped them with both Sandra and Jack Jr, scheduling appointments and making arrangements for them to get out of classes.

One week after Nurse Gallinite has gone, you receive a series of telephone messages from Mrs. Sparks. You are unable to return her calls immediately because you have recently been given a new assignment to assess the learning needs for sex education among sixth grade students. Your administrator expects a response to this analysis within 2 weeks. You plan on returning Mrs. Sparks' calls on Monday morning. Because she leaves no messages that you consider to be of a medically urgent nature, you have prioritized your time to deal with:

- An outbreak of head lice in the fourth grade classroom
- Following up on a case of suspected child abuse
- Assessing appropriate means of sex education in the sixth grade class

The telephone calls from Mrs. Sparks are initially cordial; she states that she wishes to "get to know you." As the week goes by, she calls twice each day, insisting that you call her back, that she does not have enough time to schedule appointments for her children, that she may lose her job if she does not get some help from you. Checking your messages on Thursday afternoon you find that Mrs. Sparks has called once again. On the message, she states "I guess you don't care about Jack Jr; he'll probably just go deaf if you don't start making these appointments for him."

On Friday morning, Mr. Sparks calls and speaks to you directly. He expresses anger about the fact that you have "refused" to answer his wife's calls. He informs you that the family "never had this kind of trouble with Nurse Gallinite," that she "did what the nurse is supposed to do, help the families." He accuses you of incompetence and advises you that he is going to contact your supervisor.

Questions

1) Was Nurse Gallinite a "good" school nurse? Discuss your response.

2) Were the family's expectations of you realistic? Why or why not?

3) In your role as school nurse, what does it mean to advocate for your clients?

4) Discuss the terms advocacy and empowerment as they relate to this scenario.

5) What would be an effective means of advocating for your clients in this scenario?

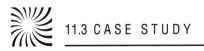 11.3 CASE STUDY

RESPONSIBILITY AND ACCOUNTABILITY IN GYNECOLOGY

SCENARIO

You are a nurse in a community health clinic. Your clinic is located in downtown Capitol City and serves an ethnically diverse, low-income population. Your client is Mary-Jo, a 36-year-old woman who has been a patient of the clinic for 15 years. She receives family planning and primary medical services at the clinic.

Mary-Jo lives with her family in a two-bedroom apartment approximately 2 miles form the clinic. She is married to Tony and together they have six children, ranging in age from 6 months to 19 years. Tony is on disability resulting from a back injury sustained on the job (long-haul trucking).

Both Mary-Jo and Tony have a long history of alcohol abuse. On several occasions Mary-Jo has asked you for information on local "detox" programs. You made several referrals and even assisted her in examining the possibility of a scholarship for an inpatient facility. Mary-Jo opted to attend Alcoholics Anonymous (AA) meetings but later informed you "I went a few times but those people are too intense for me . . . besides, I'm doing fine now." The couple's older children have had problems with truancy and have been arrested for minor infractions such as shoplifting.

Two weeks ago you received the results of Mary-Jo's most recent Pap smear, which indicated a level 4 reading. You reviewed these results with the clinic's nurse practitioner and it was decided that these results warranted immediate follow-up including a repeat Pap smear.

In the past 10 days you have spoken with Mary-Jo on seven occasions. You have discussed, in detail, the significance of the test results and strongly advised her to be seen by a physician immediately. The conversations with

Mary-Jo have taken a similar course. Your attempts at convincing, coercing, and cajoling have been met with responses about the multitude of reasons Mary-Jo is unable to make it to the clinic for follow-up. During the last conversation, Mary-Jo stated "I just don't want to come in . . . I know that those results are bad, that they could mean that I have cancer or something but I just have too much going on in my life right now to deal with anything else. I don't have anyone to watch the baby and besides, Tony takes the car every day to go out and play cards with his buddies."

Although you feel that Mary-Jo does have an understanding of the potential ramifications of her Pap smear results, she seems unwilling or unable to come to the clinic for follow-up. You do not feel that further telephone conversations will be instrumental in convincing Mary-Jo to follow up. Your supervisor has advised you that you are spending too much time on this issue and that it must come to some resolution within the next 2 days.

Questions

1) How does this scenario make you feel?

2) Discuss appropriate short- and long-term goals in this situation.
   - Short-term

   - Long-term

3) What nursing interventions would be the most beneficial for this client?
   - Immediate

   - Long-range

4) Discuss the terms autonomy and self-determination as they relate to this scenario.

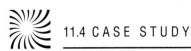 11.4 CASE STUDY

PARENTS' VERSUS CHILD'S WISHES IN TEEN PREGNANCY AND ABORTION

SCENARIO

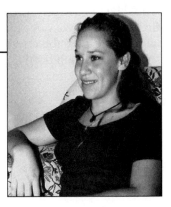

Emma is a 14-year-old student at Brownsville High School, where you work as the school nurse. You recognize Emma as a student who attended a class last month on family planning services in the community. Emma presents in your office today, Friday, at 3:00 PM. She advises you that she performed a home pregnancy test in the school bathroom this morning and that the results were positive. She asks you to assist her in telling her parents about the pregnancy. She states that she feels she would be more comfortable in your presence "because then they won't get so mad at me."

Emma states that she is "excited" about being pregnant, that she has a 17-year-old boyfriend, Randy, who "is going to make a great father . . . he'll be so excited." She adds that she "can't wait" to visit him at work today and tell him the news. Emma informs you that Randy has dropped out of school and works at a local fast food restaurant as an assistant manager. "He makes great money," she adds.

Emma lives with her parents, Jack and Josephine, in an exclusive area of Brownsville. She tells you that her parents are "great" but that they disapprove of Randy because "they think he's too old for me." She expresses concern about her mother's reaction to the pregnancy adding "I think she'll want me to have an abortion . . . she's always telling me that getting pregnant too soon would ruin my life."

Emma asks her parents to accompany her to your office on Monday morning. After she informs her parents about the pregnancy, both Jack and Josephine express anger at Emma. Josephine shouts at Emma, "We told you to use protection, we told you to go to the school clinic for birth control . . . why did you let this happen?"

The discussion remains heated despite your attempts to facilitate. Finally it is agreed that you will present the family with referrals and will meet again in a week for further discussion of the situation. You make the following referrals:

- Repeat pregnancy test by family's physician
- Family counseling services
  - Private or county

Later that week Josephine calls and asks to speak with you about Emma's "condition." She is adamant that you help her "convince" Emma to get a therapeutic abortion. She tells you that "our doctor said that it would be too dangerous for her to go through childbirth, that she's too little." She adds "we can't reason with her, she really thinks she wants this baby . . . you are the only one that she will listen to, you have to tell her that this could kill her."

Questions

1) How does it feel to be in this predicament?

2) What is your personal (not professional) response to Emma's situation?

3) As the school nurse, what are your responsibilities in this situation?

4) What actions would you take in this situation?

5) Discuss the terms advocacy and personal responsibility as they apply to this scenario.

- Advocacy

- Personal responsibility

11.5 EXERCISE

RIGHT VERSUS PRIVILEGE IN HEALTH CARE

Debate Question

Do you consider health care to be a right or a privilege?

TEAM A

Your opinion is that health care is an inherent *right*. How does your group propose to address the issues of increasing demands on limited health care resources such as funding and technology?

TEAM B

The opinion of your group is that health care is a *privilege*.
    Respond to the following questions:

1) Who should receive health care?

2) How will health care be paid for?

3) What will happen to those who desire or require health care services but are ineligible and unable to pay?

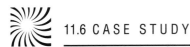 11.6 CASE STUDY

PEDIATRICS: TRANSPLANT

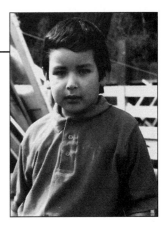

SCENARIO

You work as the client advocate for the Medicaid managed care program in Capitol City. It is 1 month before the end of your program's fiscal year. The entire staff has been advised of your program's dire financial circumstances. This is your program's second year of operations. The first year the program finished more than $450,000 in debt. Hoping to reverse that trend, the staff has focused on strict fiscal conservatism. Despite the staff's efforts, however, you have just learned that the projected deficit level for this fiscal year is well over $600,000.

You have been advised that if your program exceeds $750,000 in debt, the government is likely to revert to previous operations and eliminate the managed care program. It is generally thought that the previous method of operations was unresponsive to the needs of clients, that many clients went without needed services because of the "bureaucracy."

As the client advocate, you are contacted by Ms. Bullick who is a managed care client. Ms. Bullick tells you that she is in desperate need of your help, that a request for service has been denied by your program, and that she needs you to assist her to get what she perceives as "necessary services."

Ms. Bullick has a 7-year-old child, Alex, who has undergone two liver transplants. Although on both occasions it appeared as if the transplants were going to be successful, both were eventually rejected. Just last week Alex's physician informed Ms. Bullick that if another transplant is not performed within 4 weeks, Alex will likely die.

Ms. Bullick is a single mother. Two years ago her husband died of pancreatic cancer. Alex is an only child. One year ago Ms. Bullick quit her job as a caterer to stay home and care for Alex. She has an extremely supportive extended family living in Capitol City. Her father is active in local politics and her grandfather was mayor of the city 40 years ago.

Questions

1) Who is your client in this situation?

2) How does it feel to be in this situation?

3) Where does your primary responsibility lie?

4) What are your options? As you brainstorm, state pros and cons for each possible option.

Option	Pros	Cons

5) What do you perceive as being your best possible option?

6) What might you do on a political level to advocate for the clients you serve?

11.7 E X E R C I S E

PROS AND CONS OF AUTONOMOUS NURSING PRACTICE

Questions

1) What does the term "autonomous nursing practice" mean to you?

2) State what you perceive as the pros and cons of autonomous community health nursing practice.

Pros	Cons

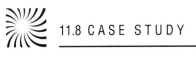 11.8 C A S E   S T U D Y

GERONTOLOGY: DEATH AND DYING

SCENARIO

You are a nurse practitioner, in private practice, specializing in gerontology. You are contracted by a network of physicians to perform home visits to their elderly clients living in rural areas surrounding Smithville.

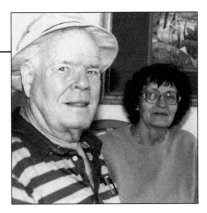

Your client is Anabelle, an 84-year-old woman who lives with Eduardo, her husband of 53 years. The couple resides in a senior citizens' apartment complex in rural Smithville. Although Anabelle has enjoyed reasonably good health throughout her life, she recently informed you, in confidence, that she feels "my time is coming soon." She is not able to provide you with specific information to back up this statement, but tells you "I have a feeling and my feelings have always been right."

Anabelle asks for your help today. She feels that she is "ready to go" but that she feels as if she is "leaving unfinished business" because she can't bring herself to talk with Eduardo about "all that doom and gloom." She vehemently adds "I don't want anything done, when it's my time," and adds "I don't want him to hook me up to one of those blasted machines." Anabelle asks you to inform both Eduardo and her physician about her feelings.

Questions

1) What does Anabelle's terminology tell you about her level of comfort with the topics of death and dying?

2) How does the term empowerment apply in this situation?

3) What are your options in this situation?

4) Given the information presented, what do you perceive as the most desirable course of action?

11.9 EXERCISE

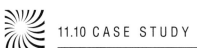

Suzanne Grant

NURSE ETHICIST

555-0001

RESOURCES FOR NURSING ETHICS

Questions

1) List resources available in your community that assist the community health nurse in analysis, interpretation, and resolution of ethical issues.
   • Agencies

   • Professional nursing organizations

   • Committees

2) How would or did you go about identifying additional resources for nursing ethics in your community?

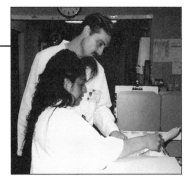

≋⦚⦚⦚⦚ 11.10 CASE STUDY

PRENATAL HIV TESTING

SCENARIO

You are a public health nurse working in a satellite prenatal clinic, on a Navajo Indian reservation, in the outskirts of Brownsville. As a result of recent information regarding the efficacy of zidovudine (AZT) prophylaxis in reducing perinatal human immunodeficiency virus (HIV) transmission, you decide that all of the clients in the prenatal satellite clinic ought to receive HIV antibody testing. In this clinic, the three public health nurses each have a caseload of clients. They are responsible for the coordination of prenatal care for these clients and see their clients during clinic days. Caseloads are determined alphabetically, with each nurse taking one-third of the alphabet.

In reviewing the charts form the clinic for your quarterly statistical report, you identify a trend in testing among the three nurses staffing the clinic:

- Nurse A (you)
  - 95% of your caseload has been educated about HIV.
  - 68% of your caseload has received HIV antibody testing.
  - 7% (one) of your clients has been identified as being HIV positive.
- Nurse B
  - 45% of the caseload has been educated about HIV.
  - 23% of the caseload has received HIV antibody testing.
  - There have been no positive test results among this group.
- Nurse C
  - 31% of the caseload has been educated about HIV.
  - 13% of the caseload has received HIV antibody testing.
  - There have been no positive test results among this group.

You feel that this is a programmatic problem with ethical implications. You decide that at the next satellite clinic staff meeting you will bring up the issue of encouraging HIV antibody testing. Present at the meeting are:

1. Three public health nurses (including yourself) who staff the clinic
2. A community health worker who lives in the Navajo community and assists in the weekly satellite clinic
3. The clinic physician, a local obstetrician whose services are contracted by the county
4. Your supervisor, the nursing director of the health department

During the course of the meeting you express your concerns and discuss the results of your data analysis regarding HIV antibody testing in the satellite clinic. Following are the responses of the group:

Physician: "The AIDS rate among these people isn't very high, its too expensive to test them all, besides we're doing better than ever before, we didn't use to test anyone."

Nurse B: "I can tell by looking at these ladies if they're in a risk group or not. Those are the ones I ask to test."

Nurse C: "It takes too much time . . . I ask them and if they say no, I say okay . . . it's their decision isn't it?"

Community health worker: "I know some of these ladies used to shoot up with drugs and some of their husbands sleep around . . . I could tell you who so you can make sure to get them tested for AIDS."

Questions

1) What are your moral and ethical responsibilities in this matter?

2) What would you like to see happen:
   - In the meeting

   - In the clinics

3) What are the responsibilities of the following parties in this scenario:
   - Your employer, the health department

   - Your supervisor

   - Clinic physician

   - Your fellow nurses

   - Community health worker

- The clients

4) If no change results from this meeting, what recourse do you have?

- What actions would you take?

References

Bishop, N. J., & Goldie, S. (1962). *A Bio-bibliography of Florence Nightingale*. London: International Council of Nurses.

Davis, A., & Aroskar, M. (1978). *Ethical dilemmas and nursing practice*. New York: Appleton-Century-Crofts.

Webster's II new Riverside University dictionary. (1984). Boston: The Riverside Publishing Company, A Houghton Mifflin Company.

CHAPTER 12

The Global Influence of the Community Health Nurse: Research, Development, and Political Involvement

"Talent is nurtured in solitude; character is formed in the stormy billows of the world."

Goethe

Political involvement, policy development, and nursing research are issues that affect all nurses. Chapter 12 highlights the roles and responsibilities of community health nurses in each of these areas.

REVIEW

I. Research
   A. Research question
   B. Research design
   C. Data collection
   D. Data analysis
   E. Data interpretation
   F. Disseminating information
   G. Types of research
      1. Qualitative

      2. Quantitative
      3. Experimental
      4. Nonexperimental
   H. Use of technology in nursing research
    I. Legal and ethical issues related to nursing research
  II. Program planning and policy development
    A. Funding sources
    B. Program evaluation
    C. History of nursing's role in planning and health care policy
      1. Florence Nightingale
      2. Lillian Wald and Mary Brewster
    D. Health care planning
      1. Local
      2. State
      3. National
      4. International
    E. Policy development
      1. Analysis of existing policies
      2. Political involvement
        a) Individual
        b) Group
        c) Professional
          (1) Nursing's power
III. Political involvement
    A. Professional nursing organizations
    B. Personal political action
    C. Review of legislative process
    D. Levels of political activity

DISCUSSION

Research

Although research has been used by nurses to delineate boundaries of existing roles, it may also be used to identify new possibilities, new roles for nurses. Research, particularly in the environment of health care reform, will afford nurses opportunities to identify new and more effective methods of nursing intervention.

    Nurses have long been affected by the influence of increasing expectations for positive outcomes complicated by fiscal constraints. Nursing, therefore, is uniquely qualified to initiate research that addresses these issues as they relate to managed care.

    With a decrease in available funding for all health care services, it is incumbent on nursing to justify its existence in the age of health care reform. Nurses must demonstrate their value in terms of both cost effectiveness and optimal client outcomes. Nursing research is the means to this end.

Theory development in community health nursing involves the definition of concepts and testing of hypotheses as well as other types of research. The focus areas of this research include:

- Aggregates
  - Pregnant women
  - Elderly
  - Cultural groups
- Practice settings
  - Home health
  - Public health
- Specialty areas
  - Administration
  - Education
- Programs
  - Quarterly reports for grant funded programs

Policy Development and Political Action

Although nurses are greatly affected by legislation and policy related to the provision of health care, they are sorely underrepresented in the developmental process of such policies. Nurses have joined forces to advocate for their clients and their profession. The fact remains, however, that many of the policy and planning decisions that affect the nursing profession are made by such nonnurses as hospital administrators, politicians, and physician groups. Public health nurses, as the largest group of health care professionals delivering public health services, are charged with providing leadership that will work to ensure equitable distribution of available resources to meet the needs of the community (McKnight & Van Dover, 1994, p. 12).

Nurses must continue to participate politically on all levels, personally and professionally, and must continue to search for new ways of having their voices heard. Change, such as that anticipated with reform of the health care system, presents nursing with an opportunity to establish new roles in the areas of planning and policy development. For nursing to present a powerful force in the development of health care policy, the profession must identify mutual goals along with methods and resources that maximize the profession's potential to work collaboratively to effect change.

Political Activity

Figure 12-1 (Hanley, 1984, p. 302) represents the various levels of political activity

Program Planning

The nursing process may be used to assist the nurse in program planning. Following are examples of specific activities for the components of the nursing process.

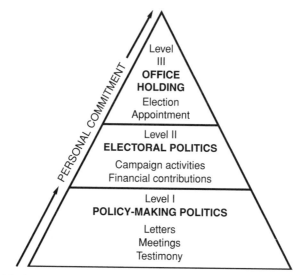

FIGURE 12-1 The levels of political activity. Adapted from Hanley (1984, p. 302).

I. Assessment
   A. Qualitative and quantitative data
      1. Vital statistics
      2. Demographics
      3. Population
      4. Environmental
      5. Socioeconomic
      6. Health care services and utilization
II. Statement of problems
   A. Interpret above information and cite evidence of problems
   B. Indicate populations affected
III. Plan
   A. Analyze existing public policy related to issues (how do these policies impact the problem?)
   B. Identify resources to achieve desired outcomes
   C. Cost–benefit analysis
   D. Educational approaches
IV. Implementation
   A. Three levels of implementation (DeBella, Martin, & Siddall, 1986, p. 39)
      1. "Public policy-making—converts a planning proposal into legislation and regulations
      2. Administrative adoption of the planned interventions—creates the organizations to carry out the programs that have been legislated
      3. Operations—obtains the suitable responses and participation from those who are part of the implementation effort, or who are affected by the interventions"

V. Evaluation
   A. Must include
      1. Outcomes of change
      2. Positive
      3. Negative
      4. Cost of change
      5. Impact of change on delivery of health care
      6. Impact on profession of nursing

Case Studies and Exercises

Responses to the following case studies and exercises reflect the ability to:

1. Participate in political strategies to enhance the public's perception of nursing and health care issues.
2. Analyze the impact of health care policies on clients.
3. Frame a research question.
4. Outline a plan to "sell" others on a particular policy or program.
5. Give examples of personal and professional involvement at the various levels of political activity.
6. Differentiate between issues warranting political action and policy change.

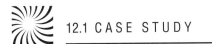

12.1 CASE STUDY

PEDIATRICS: HEALTH PROMOTION

SCENARIO

You work as the assistant director of nursing in the Brownsville Health Center. The mayor, who was recently elected, ran on the slogan "our children are our future." This was in response to public sentiment that the health and welfare of the community's children had declined in recent years.

    Shortly after his election, the mayor approached the health officer and director of nursing for the county health department. He asked for their assistance in increasing the health of the children of Brownsville. "We want everyone to start thinking about children's health," he informed them. "I don't want any of our children to be without health services." Although the mayor seems to feel that additional services are needed for the children of Brownsville, he balks at the discussion of additional funding for programs or services.

After an in-depth review of existing programs, you and your supervisor, the nursing director, identify numerous services offered through the health department aimed at promoting the health of Brownsville's children.

Examples of such services include:

- Immunization clinics, mobile and satellite
- Satellite well-baby clinics
- Medicaid managed care coverage for services such as prenatal care, well-baby care, and pediatric illness coverage
- Health education programs on child safety and parenting

In comparing health indicators of your population, you identify the following:

1. Infant mortality, 3% lower than the state average
2. Immunization rate, 5% higher than the state average
3. Rate of childhood injury attributable to motor vehicle accidents, 17% higher than national average
4. Few educational programs for developmentally disabled children

Questions

1) What other indices related to children's health will you evaluate?

2) What do you think about the perception, on the part of both the public and the mayor, that the health needs of Brownsville's children are not being adequately addressed?

3) What do you think about the mayor's request for sweeping program and policy change?

4) Plan a comprehensive strategy to increase public awareness of existing services.

12.2 E X E R C I S E

RESEARCH

You are a student in a master's of nursing program. As part of your coursework, you are to discuss ways in which you will develop a research strategy to analyze the following issue:

Impact on infant mortality among Medicaid clients in Capitol City since the inception of Medicaid managed care

Questions

1) How will you frame your research question, giving consideration to the following issues:
   - Population

   - Hypothesis

   - Variables

   - Data

   - Indices to be measured

2) What resources will you use to assist you in your research?

12.3 E X E R C I S E

CONTRACT BID

SCENARIO

You are the nurse educator/quality assurance supervisor for a home health agency in Brownsville. Your agency is competing for a local managed care contract to provide home health services to the Medicaid and Medicare populations.

- List data you will use to support your agency in its bid for this contract.

- List information about your agency that would convince the managed care organization to grant your agency the contract (assume that the services you deem valuable are offered by your agency).

- Present supporting data related to:
  - Cost containment

  - Client satisfaction

  - Positive health outcomes

  - Other

12.4 EXERCISE

POLICY CHANGE

SCENARIO

As an independent nurse practitioner and certified nurse midwife, you perceive a need for policy change on the state level regarding licensure for midwives. Currently lay midwives and certified midwives have equal privileges under county-operated managed care guidelines. You feel that your scope of practice is limited because of the existing policy that does not 'panel' or reimburse midwives for prenatal or delivery services. You feel strongly that by reimbursing certified nurse midwives the managed care program could provide high-quality cost-effective services to clients, many of whom experience difficulty obtaining prenatal care services.

Discuss the steps you will take to bring your concept of necessary policy change through the following phases:

• Community organization

• Professional support

• Legislative support

12.5 EXERCISE

POLITICAL INVOLVEMENT IN YOUR COMMUNITY

What is the level of political involvement by and for nurses in your community?

Respond to the following questions. If unable to answer, provide ideas about potential resources in your community to obtain information related to the issue.

Questions

1) What opportunities exist for registered nurses in your community to become involved in politically active professional nursing organizations?

2) At your school or employing agency, what types of support and mentorship are available to you?

3) Discuss political representation by nurses in your community.

4) Think of a health-related issue that you feel warrants additional attention by community leaders (ie, nursing positions, AIDS education, etc).
   - What steps will you take to voice your personal opinion regarding this issue?

   - How will you go about effecting change, related to this issue, in your community?

12.6 EXERCISE

POLITICAL ACTION

Each member of the group or class responds to the following questions by writing anonymously on corresponding sheet of paper placed throughout the room.

Question

1) How do you stay informed about political actions affecting the following:
   - Federal, state, and local laws

   - Your profession

   - Your area of practice/specialty area

   - Your clients

   - Your community

   Review and discuss the group's responses.
   In your opinion, what are the responsibilities of the professional nurse related to political involvement?

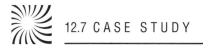 12.7 CASE STUDY

GOVERNMENTAL BUDGETARY DECISIONS AND RESPONSE TO SPENDING CUTS

SCENARIO

The federal government, in an effort to reduce the deficit, has decided to cut several social programs. The free school lunch program is one program targeted for elimination. The proposal is to replace the free school lunch program with an increase of $12 per month per child in AFDC checks to families. The government claims that families will spend the extra $12 on lunches for their children. It is estimated that this will save the federal government over $1 million dollars in the cost of administering the program.

Respond to this fictitious scenario given the following requests:

As a member of a professional organization of school nurses, you have been asked by the group to:

- Identify probable ramifications of the proposed actions

- Develop alternative approaches to cost savings in the school lunch program (a farm subsidy program)

12.8 EXERCISE

POLITICAL ACTION: SCOPE OF PRACTICE

SCENARIO

You are a member of a statewide professional group of home health nurses. Your group has voiced concern about the following issues that are affecting their scope of practice:

1. Increasing use of home health aides to perform skilled tasks
2. Overwhelming documentation requirements for Medicaid and Medicare
3. Poor perception of the role of the home health nurse by the general public as well as local politicians

4. Number of home visits reimbursed by Medicaid, Medicare, and most managed care organizations inadequate to ensure quality
5. Home health nursing services (education, prevention, etc)

Which of the above issues warrant:

• Political action

• Policy change

12.9 EXERCISE

FUNDING AND POLICY

SCENARIO

With block grant funding, states will administer Medicaid money. Previously, Medicaid funding was provided by the federal government. Discuss effective means of fiscal management with block grant funding given the following information:

• You are a nurse serving on the governor's health care task force.
• Funding available: $10,000,000
• Health care budget from last year
  ○ 23% acute care services
  ○ 14% prescription medications
  ○ 18% skilled nursing facilities
  ○ 12% private physicians
  ○ 5% primary care
  ○ 9% specialists
  ○ 8% mental health services
  ○ 5% home health services
  ○ 4% developmentally disabled
  ○ 2% preventive services

Question

1) What recommendations will you make in your role as a member on the governor's task force?

- What specific information will you need?

- How will you obtain this information?

- How will you determine if the needs of the population are being met?

References

DeBella, S., Martin, L., & Siddall, S. (1986). *Nurses' role in health care planning*. Norwalk, CT: Appleton-Century-Crofts.

Hanley, B. (1984). Legislation and policy. In Sullivan, J. (Ed.). *Directions in community health nursing* (pp. 293–317). Cambridge, MA: Blackwell Scientific Publications.

McKnight, J., & Van Dover, L. (1994). Community as client: A challenge for nursing education. *Public Health Nursing, 11*(1), 12–16.

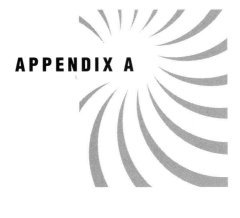

APPENDIX A

Suggested Readings
by Content Area

Autonomy

Schutzenhofer, K., & Musser, D. (1994). Nurse characteristics and professional autonomy. *Image: Journal of Nursing Scholarship, 26*(3), 201–206.

Caregivers

Boland, D., & Sims, S. (1996). Family care giving at home as a solitary journey. *Image: Journal of Nursing Scholarship, 28*(1), 55–58.

England, M. (1996). Content domain for caregiver planning identified by adult offspring caregivers. *Image: Journal of Nursing Scholarship, 28*(1), 17–22.

Case Management

Beresford, L. (1991). Cracking the big case. *Case Manager, 2*(3), 50–58.

Bigelow, D., & Young, D. (1991). Effectiveness of a case management program. *Community Mental Health Journal, 27*(2), 115–122.

Engen, C. (1995). A permanent commission for certified case managers. *Journal of Care Management, 1*(2), 19.

Goering, P., Wasylenki, D., Onge, M., Paduchak, D., & Lancee, W. (1992). Gender differences among clients of a case management program for the homeless. *Hospital and Community Psychiatry, 43*(2), 160–165.

Goodwin, D. (1994). Nursing case management activities: How they differ between employment settings. *Journal of Nursing Administration, 24*(2), 29–34.

Hogue, E. (1995). Are case managers liable? *Journal of Care Management, 1*(2), 35–50.

Moffat, J. (1991). Case management in a managed care environment. *Case Manager, 2*(3), 64–75.

Rheaume, A., Frisch, S., & Kennedy, C. (1994). Case management and nursing practice. *Journal of Nursing Administration, 24*(3), 30–36.

Rothman, J. (1991). A model of case management: Toward empirically based practice. *Social Work, 36*(6), 520–528.

Community as Client

Barker, J., Bayne, T., Higgs, Z., Jenkin, S., Murphy, D., & Synoground, G. (1994). Community analysis: A collaborative community practice project. *Public Health Nursing, 11*(2), 104–112.

McKnight, J., & Van Dover, L. (1994). Community as client: A challenge for nursing education. *Public Health Nursing, 11*(1), 12–16.

Community Health Nursing (General)

de la Cruz, F. (1994). Clinical decision making styles of home healthcare nurses. *Image: Journal of Nursing Scholarship, 26*(3), 222–226.

Hamilton, P., & Keyser, P. (1992). The relationship of ideology to developing community health nursing theory. *Public Health Nursing, 9*(3), 142–148.

Stevens, P., & Hall, J. (1992). Applying critical theories to nursing in communities. *Public Health Nursing, 9*(1), 2–9.

Sullivan, J. (Ed.). (1984). *Directions in community health nursing*. Cambridge, MA: Blackwell Scientific Publications.

Culture

Carney, P. (1992). The concept of poverty. *Public Health Nursing, 9*(2), 74–80.

Environment of Care

Clarke, Pl., & Cody, W. (1994). Nursing theory–based practice in the home and community: The crux of professional nursing education. *Advances in Nursing Science, 17*(2), 41–53.

Davis, J., & Deitrick, E. (1988). Novice home visitors teaching/learning needs. *Public Health Nursing, 5*(4), 214–218.

Liaschenko, J. (1994). The moral geography of home care. *Advances in Nursing Science, 17*(2), 16–26.

O'Neil, E. (1994). Home health nurses' use of base rate information in diagnostic reasoning. *Advances in Nursing Science, 17*(2), 77–85.

Hospice

Bailey, B. (1990). The concepts of empowerment and care of the hospice patient and family. *Journal of Home Health Care Practice, 3*(1), 16–22.

Gentile, M., & Fello, M. (1990). Hospice care for the 1990s: A concept coming of age. *Journal of Home Health Care Practice, 3*(1), 1–15.

Kübler-Ross, E. (1969). *On death and dying*. New York: Macmillan.

Policy, Planning, and Politics

DeBella, S., Martin, L., & Siddall, S. (1986). Nurses' role in health care planning. Norwalk, CT: Appleton-Century-Crofts.

Locke, L., Spirduso, W., & Silverman, S. (1988). *Proposals that work: A guide for planning dissertations and grant proposals* (2nd ed.). Newbury Park, CA: Sage.

Thomas, P., & Shelton, C. (1994). Teaching students to become active in public policy. *Public Health Nursing, 11*(2), 75–79.

Psychiatric and Mental Health

Feldman, R., & Kocin, M. (1991). Caring for disoriented clients with Alzheimer's disease at home. *Journal of Home Health Care Practice, 3*(4), 40–47.

Reinhard, S. (1994). Perspectives on the family's caregiving experience in mental illness. *Image: Journal of Nursing Scholarship, 26*(1), 70–74.

Simms, C. (1995). How to unmask the angry patient. *American Journal of Nursing, 95*(4), 37–40.

Quality Assurance

Carefoote, R. (1994). Total quality management implementation in home care agencies. *Journal of Nursing Administration, 24*(10), 31–37.

Klug, R. (1994). Setting home care standards. *Pediatric Nursing, 20*(4), 404–406.

Sherman, J., & Malkmus, M. (1994). Integrating quality assurance and total quality management/quality improvement. *Journal of Nursing Administration, 24*(3), 37–41.

Tahan, H., & Cesta, T. (1994). Developing case management plans using a quality improvement model. *Journal of Nursing Administration, 24*(12), 49–58.

Zlotnick, C. (1992). A public health quality assurance system. *Public Health Nursing, 9*(2), 133–137.

Research

Bard, J., Jimenez, F., & Tornack, R. (1994). An outcome-focused, community-based health support program. *Journal of Nursing Administration, 24*(3), 48–54.

Rural and International Health

Dansky, K. (1995). The impact of healthcare reform on rural home health agencies. *Journal of Nursing Administration, 25*(3), 27–33.

Werner, D. (1983). *Where there is no doctor: A village health care handbook.* Palo Alto, CA: The Hesperian Foundation.

Werner, D., & Bower, B. (1983). *Helping health workers learn.* Palo Alto, CA: The Hesperian Foundation.

Safety

Carter, S., Carrol, M., & Hayes, E. (1994). Environmental safety preparation for community-based nursing educational experiences: Measurable indices. *Public Health Nursing, 11*(5), 300–304.

Zerwekh, J. (1991). At the expense of their souls. *Nursing Outlook, 39*(2), 58–61.

Trends

Aiken, L., & Salmon, M. (1994). Health care workforce priorities: What nursing should do now. *Inquiry, 31,* 318–329.

Feingold, E. (1994). Health care reform—More than cost containment and universal access. *American Journal of Public Health, 84*(5), 727–728.

Huch, M. (1995). Nursing and the next millennium. *Nursing Science Quarterly, 8*(1), 38–44.

Johnson, J. (1995). Curricular trends in accredited generic baccalaureate nursing programs across the United States. *Journal of Nursing Education, 34*(2), 53–60.

Knollmueller, R. (1994). Thinking about tomorrow for nursing: Changes and challenges. *Journal of Continuing Education in Nursing, 25*(5), 196–201.

Manion, J. (1995). Understanding the seven stages of change. *American Journal of Nursing, 95*(4), 41–43.

Wolf, G., Boland, S., & Aukerman, M. (1994). A transformational model for the practice of professional nursing: Part 1, the model. *Journal of Nursing Administration, 24*(4), 51–57.

Wolf, G., Boland, S., & Aukerman, M. (1994). A transformational model for the practice of professional nursing: Part 2. *Journal of Nursing Administration, 24*(5), 38–46.

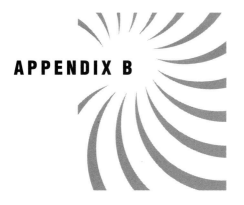

APPENDIX B

Professional Resources

Caregiver Resources

Alzheimer's Association
(800) 262-3900

Alzheimer's Disease and Education Referral Center
(800) 438-4380

American Association of Homes and Services for the Aging
(202) 783-2242

American Association of Retired Persons
(202) 434-2277

American Orthotic and Prosthetic Association
(703) 836-7118

Assisted Living Facilities Association of America
(703) 692-8100

Eldercare Locator, National Association of Area Agencies on Aging
(800) 677-1116

National Hospice Organization
PO Box 9998
Arlington, VA 22209
(800) 658-8898

National Information Center for Children and Youth with Handicaps
PO Box 1492
Washington, DC 20013
(703) 893-6061

National Institute on Aging
(301) 496-1752

National Mental Health Association
(800) 969-6642

Case Management

CERTIFICATION

CIRSC/Certified Case Manager
1835 Rohlwing Road, Suite D
Rolling Meadows, IL 60008
(708) 818-0292

GENERAL

The Center for Case Management
6 Pleasant Street
South Natick, MA 01760

Individual Case Management Association
11830 Westline Industrial Drive
St. Louis, MO 63146
(800) 664-2620

Case Management Society of America
1101 17th Street, N.W., Suite 1200
Washington, DC 20036
(202) 296-9200

The National Association of Professional Geriatric Care Managers
655 North Alvernon Way, Suite 108
Tucson, AZ 85711

National Coalition of Associations for the Advancement of Case Management
20953 Devonshire Street, Suite 2
Chatsworth, CA 91311
(818) 407-0478

Health Insurance

American Health Information Management Association
919 North Michigan Avenue, Suite 1400
Chicago, IL 60611
(312) 787-2672

American Managed Care and Review Association
1227 25th Street, N.W., Suite 610
Washington, DC 20037
(202) 728-0506

Blue Cross and Blue Shield Association
676 North Saint Clair Street
Chicago, IL 60610
(312) 440-5526

Health Insurance Association of America
1025 Connecticut Avenue, N.W.
Washington, DC 20036-3998
(202) 223-7780

Managed Healthcare News (publication)
(800) 949-6525

National Insurance Consumer Helpline
(800) 942-4242

The Health Care Cost Hotline
(800) 225-2500

"Your Medicare Handbook"
Free by calling (800) 638-6833
Also available at local Social Security offices

Home Care

Visiting Nurse Association of America
3801 East Florida Avenue, Suite 900
Denver, CO 80210

National Association for Home Care
228 7th Street, S.E.
Washington, DC, 20003

American Academy of Home Care Physicians
4550 West 77th Street, Suite 100
Edina, MN 55435
(612) 835-1972

National Association for Home Care
519 C Street, N.E.
Washington, DC 20002
(202) 547-3540

Hospice

Hospice Association of America
228 7th Street, S.E.
Washington, DC 20003

Public Health

American Public Health Association
1015 15th Street, N.W., Suite 300
Washington, DC 20005

The Healthcare Forum
(Tools for creating healthier communities)
(415) 356-4300

Quality Assurance

InterQual CM/UM criteria (publication)
44 Lafayette Road
PO Box 988
North Hampton, NH 03862
(603) 964-7255

National Committee for Quality Assurance (NCQA)
1350 York Avenue, N.W., Suite 700
Washington, DC 20005
(202) 628-5788

School Nursing

American School Health Association
7263 State Route 43
Kent, OH 44240

National Association of School Nurses
PO Box 1300
Scarborough, ME 04070

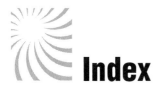

Index

Note: Page numbers followed by *f* indicate figures; those followed by *t* indicate tables.